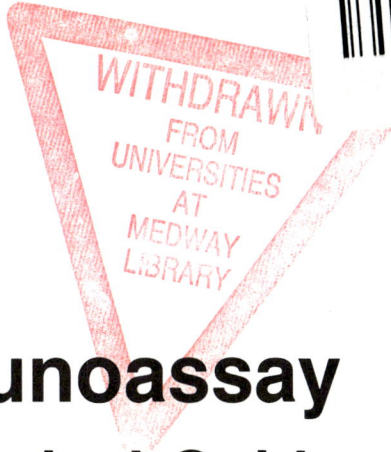

Immunoassay
A Practical Guide

Edited by

Daniel W. Chan

Department of Laboratory Medicine
Clinical Chemistry Division
The Johns Hopkins Hospital
Johns Hopkins University
Baltimore, Maryland

Associate Editor

Marie T. Perlstein

Ortho Pharmaceuticals
Raritan, New Jersey

1987

ACADEMIC PRESS, INC.

Harcourt Brace Jovanovich, Publishers
Orlando   San Diego   New York   Austin
Boston   London   Sydney   Tokyo   Toronto

ACADEMIC PRESS, INC.
Orlando, Florida 32887

United Kingdom Edition published by
ACADEMIC PRESS INC. (LONDON) LTD.
24–28 Oval Road, London NW1 7DX

Library of Congress Cataloging in Publication Data

Immunoassay : a practical guide.

Includes index.
1. Immunoassay.   I. Chan, Daniel W. (Daniel Wan-Yui)
II. Perlstein, Marie T.   [DNLM: 1. Immunoassay—methods.
QW 570 I325]
RB46.5.I423   1987   616.07′56   87-1771
ISBN 0–12–167635–8 (alk. paper)

PRINTED IN THE UNITED STATES OF AMERICA

87 88 89 90   9 8 7 6 5 4 3 2 1

Contents

4. Clinical Validation of Immunoassays: A Well-Designed Approach to a Clinical Study

Mark H. Zweig and E. Arthur Robertson

5. Data Reduction Techniques for Immunoassay

George F. Johnson

6. Immunoassays: Quality Control and Troubleshooting

Marie T. Perlstein

Preface

During the last few years, immunoassay has gained tremendous popularity in clinical and research laboratories and has been applied to determine hormone, enzyme, protein, drug, and infectious agent.

The advent of monoclonal antibodies allows for measurement of analytes by immunoassay that were previously difficult to analyze. In some instances, immunoassay has replaced "traditional" methods, for example, the measurement of enzyme mass rather than enzyme activity and the determination of drug concentration by immunoassay rather than chromatography.

Most published books in immunoassay deal with the theory or the method for a specific analyte. Few books discuss the practical aspects of immunoassay. This book is based on workshop materials given by a number of the contributors during the last ten years to various professional societies, including the American Association for Clinical Chemistry (AACC), American Society for Clinical Pathology (ASCP), American Society for Medical Technology (ASMT), and Clinical Ligand Assay Society (CLAS).

The aim of this book is to provide clinical laboratory personnel and students with an understanding of the principle of immunoassay (Chapter 1) and the production of reagents for immunoassay (Chapter 2). With the availability of commercial reagents and immunoassay "kits," it is important for laboratory personnel to use good judgment in the selection of an immunoassay method. Chapters 3 and 4 provide such a practical guide for assessing the analytical and clinical performances of immunoassay. Chapter 5 provides an understanding of the data reduction method as well as some practical computer programs. Chapter 6 provides a quality control program and recommendations for troubleshooting.

We would like to thank the editorial office at Academic Press for support in the publication of this book.

Daniel W. Chan
Marie T. Perlstein

Chapter 1

General Principle of Immunoassay

Daniel W. Chan

Department of Laboratory Medicine
Clinical Chemistry Division
The Johns Hopkins Hospital
and School of Medicine
Johns Hopkins University
Baltimore, Maryland 21205

I. INTRODUCTION

A. Principle of Analytical Techniques

The determination of a substance in biological fluid usually consists of at least two steps—reaction and detection. The nature of the reaction and the detection steps can be physical, chemical, biological, or immunological (Table I).

Immunoassay involves the binding of antigen to antibody, followed by a physical separation of this "bound" antigen from the "unbound" antigen in the heterogeneous system. However, homogeneous immunoassay requires no physical separation. The detection system can be a radioactive label with a radioactive counter for radioimmunoassay (RIA), an enzyme label with a spectrophotometer for enzyme immunoassay (EIA), or a fluorescent label with a fluorometer for fluorescence immunoassay (FIA).

The binder in the assay system may not have to be an antibody. In the receptor assay, the binder is a receptor. The radioreceptor assay for pregnancy testing uses a receptor for human chorionic gonadotropin (hCG), for example, Biocept-G, the once popular radioreceptor assay (RRA) manufactured by Wampole Laboratory (Saxena *et al.*, 1974). This assay is not specific for hCG because lutropin (LH) with a similar α subunit also cross-reacts with the receptor. In the com-

Table I. Comparison of Analytical Methods[a]

Parameter	Heterogeneous immunoassay	Homogeneous immunoassay	Chromatographic method	Chemical method
Specificity	+	0	+	−
Sensitivity	+ +	+	0	−
Precision	+	+ +	+	+ +
Multiple analytes	− −	− −	+ +	0
Automation	0	+	0	+ +
Analysis time	−	+	−	−
Technical expertise	0	+	− −	+ +
Cost				
Reagent/disposable	−	− −	+ +	+ +
Instrumentation	+	0	− −	+
Correlation with				
bioactivity	0	0	0	0

[a] +, Advantage; −, disadvantage; 0, average.

petitive protein binding assay (CPBA), a naturally occurring protein in plasma is used instead of an antibody. For example, thyroxine-binding globulin (TBG) is used in the competitive protein binding assay to measure thyroxine (T_4); cortisol-binding globulin (CBG) or transcortin is used in the CPBA to measure cortisol. The radioassay for folate uses a milk binder and the assay for vitamin B_{12} uses intrinsic factor (IF).

The heterogeneous immunoassay with a separation step usually involves centrifugation or washing the antigen–antibody complex to remove unbound antigen. This separation step also removes other interfering substances in the sample. Therefore, it tends to be more specific than a corresponding homogeneous immunoassay. Furthermore, its sensitivity can be better as a result of less interference. However, heterogeneous immunoassay requires more manipulations, for instance, a washing–separation step and an enzyme–substrate reaction step. The precision tends to be less than in a homogeneous immunoassay, especially if the homogeneous assay is automated. Automation is simpler and easier for homogeneous immunoassay, and the analysis time is shorter. Examples of such homogeneous immunoassays for therapeutic drug monitoring (TDM) are a fluorescent polarization immunoassay (FPIA) on the TDx analyzer manufactured by Abbott Laboratories and an enzyme immunoassay, the Syva EMIT (enzyme multiplied immunoassay technique), on the Roche Cobas-Bio analyzer. Immunoassays usually measure only one analyte at a time. Multiple analytes such as a drug and its metabolites cannot be analyzed in a single run. The technical expertise needed in performing immunoassays has been changing during the past decade. Dedicated personnel were once a requirement for performing RIA. Now, the automated homogeneous immunoassay can be performed by almost any trained laboratory personnel. The cost of homogeneous immunoassay reagents, though decreasing as there is more competition between manufacturers, is still greater than that of reagents for heterogeneous immunoassays. In addition, the instrumentation cost to perform heterogeneous immunoassays is lower; in most instances, a simple spectrophotometer or colorimeter is sufficient.

In chromatographic technique, the separation of an analyte from other substances is achieved by a chromatographic column using liquid–liquid interaction, as in high-performance liquid chromatography (HPLC), or gas–liquid interaction, as in gas–liquid chromatography (GLC). Then the analyte can be detected by using an ultraviolet (UV), fluorescence, electrochemical, or refractive index detector. In a gas–liquid chromatography–mass spectrometry (GC-MS) system, the separation step is GC and the detection step is MS. Most chromatographic methods are specific. Each analyte can be identified by its characteristic retention time in the column. Although the absolute recovery through extraction and chromatographic steps is generally poor, the relative recovery with the use of internal standard and calibrators provides consistent quantitative determination. These methods have been applied almost exclusively to the determination of small analytes, as in the analysis of drugs. Recently, large molecules such as proteins and enzymes have been analyzed successfully by HPLC. The sensitivity of chromatographic techniques is less than that of immunoassay. A good example is digoxin. The method of choice for its analysis for many years has been RIA because the chromatographic methods are not sensitive down to nanogram concentrations. Improved sensitivity in GC can be achieved by using a more sensitive detection system, such as a nitrogen–phosphorus or an electron capture detector. The greatest advantage of chromatography is the ability to determine multiple analytes in the same analytical run. Simultaneous determinations of four anticonvulsants by GC (Least et al., 1975), six anticonvulsants by HPLC (Adams and Vandemark, 1976), and 12 common sedatives and hypnotics by HPLC (Kabra et al., 1978) have been reported. Automation is usually at the sample injection step. Sequential analysis of one sample at a time is inefficient, particularly with a large batch of samples. Chromatography generally requires highly trained personnel. This may be the reason why therapeutic drug monitoring was not widely performed in clinical laboratories until immunoassays become available. Reagents for chromatography usually consist of inexpensive organic solvents. However, instruments can be costly, for example, for GC-MS.

The chemical method involves either chemical reaction or enzymatic reaction followed by measurement with a spectrophotometer or fluorometer. In general, chemical methods are less sensitive and specific than the other methods and are subject to a variety of interferences. However, they are relatively easy to automate.

Each technique is suitable for analyzing certain substances. Traditionally, radioimmunoassay has been used to measure hormone concentrations in serum or urine. More recently, two-sites (sandwich) immunoradiometric assay has been used to measure polypeptide hormones. Nonisotopic immunoassay with an enzyme or fluorescent label is being used in the clinical laboratory, especially in therapeutic drug monitoring. Examples are the EMIT reagent by Syva and the TDx reagent by Abbott. Nonisotopic immunoassay not only eliminates radioactivity but also offers a greater potential for automation with existing instrumentation in the clinical laboratory. It improves the efficiency of test analysis.

B. Classification of Immunoassays

Immunoassays can be classified according to two different approaches: competitive immunoassay, such as radioimmunoassay (RIA), and immunometric assay, such as immunoradiometric assay (IRMA) and immunoenzymetric assay (IEMA).

1. Competitive Immunoassay

In the competitive immunoassay approach, which is also termed the "labeled analyte" technique (Ekins, 1981), there exists a competition of the unlabeled antigen with labeled antigen (e.g., radioactively labeled antigen) for a limited amount of binding sites on the binder (e.g., antibody) (Fig. 1). Traditional RIA uses this approach. Only a small amount of antibody is required for RIA. The assay can be performed by adding the antigen and antibody simultaneously or sequentially. Although most RIA is performed simultaneously, sequential assay with incubation of the antibody with the sample before adding labeled antigen may improve the sensitivity of the assay.

2. Immunometric Assay

In the immunometric assay approach, which is also termed the "labeled reagent" technique (Ekins, 1981), an excess amount of labeled binder, such as antibody, is present to extract antigen (Fig. 2). Single labeled antibody can be

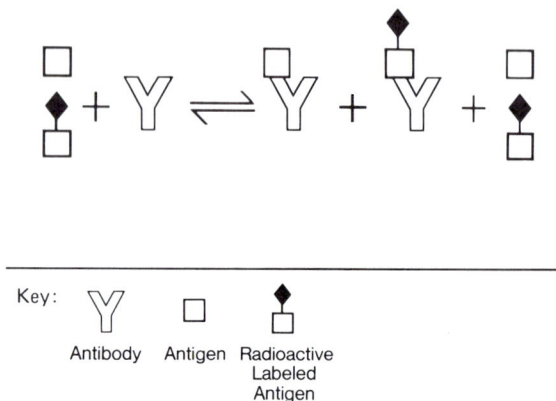

Figure 1. Competitive immunoassay: radioimmunoassay (RIA).

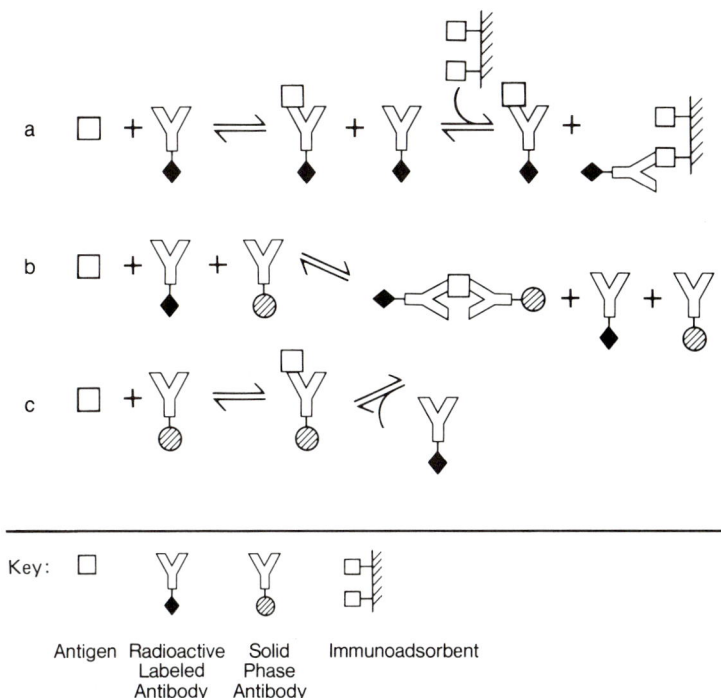

Figure 2. Immunometric assay: immunoradiometric assay (IRMA). a, Single labeled antibody technique; b, simultaneous "sandwich" IRMA; and c, sequential "sandwich" IRMA.

used to bind antigen. Then the excess "unbound" labeled antibody can be removed by an absorbent. Two antibodies, one labeled and the other unlabeled but attached to a solid support, can be used to form a binding complex with the antigen—a "sandwich." A limitation of the two-site immunometric assay has been the need for large amounts of antibodies. With the advances in monoclonal antibody techniques, large-scale production of antibodies can be achieved. Another disadvantage of this system is the "high-dose hook" effect: when a large amount of antigen is present, antibody concentration becomes a limiting factor. The immunoassay reaction behaves like a traditional competitive assay; therefore, the response is no longer linear. This is particularly troublesome for analyte with wide concentration ranges, e.g., tumor marker. The concentration of AFP seen in patients with hepatocellular carcinoma varies from ng/ml to mg/ml (Chan et al., 1986). However, the immunometric assay offers good sensitivity and short incubation times. This technique can be applied only to polypeptide antigens with at least two distinct antibody binding sites. It is ideal for polypeptide hormones and tumor markers, such as carcinoembryonic antigen (CEA), α-fetoprotein (AFP), and chorionic gonadotropin (hCG), but not for small molecules such as drugs, triiodothyronine (T_3), and T_4.

II. THEORETICAL BASIS OF IMMUNOASSAY

A. Basic Assumptions

The following assumptions are required in order to develop a mathematical model for competitive immunoassay (Campfield, 1983).

1. The antigen is present in homogeneous form, consisting of only one chemical species.
2. The antibody is also present in one homogeneous chemical form.
3. Both antigen and antibody are univalent; i.e., one molecule of antigen can react with one molecule of antibody.
4. Labeled and unlabeled antigens have similar physical–chemical properties.
5. The antigen–antibody reaction is governed by the law of mass action, assuming no allosteric or cooperative effects are present.
6. The reaction reaches equilibrium.
7. Separation of bound and free antigen is perfect and does not disturb the equilibrium.
8. The ratio of bound to free antigen or the ratio of bound to total antigen can be measured perfectly.

B. Scatchard Plot

The immunoassay reaction can be described by the Scatchard plot (Scatchard, 1949), based on

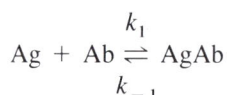

$$\text{Ag} + \text{Ab} \underset{k_{-1}}{\overset{k_1}{\rightleftharpoons}} \text{AgAb}$$

where Ag is the antigen, Ab the antibody, AgAB the antigen–antibody complex, k_1 the association rate constant, and k_{-1} the dissociation rate constant.

At equilibrium,

$$K = k_1/k_{-1} = (\text{AgAb})/(\text{Ag})(\text{Ab})$$

where K is the affinity constant, and

$$b/f = (\text{AgAb})/(\text{Ag}) = K(\text{Ab})$$
$$b/f = K(\text{Ab}_T - B)$$

where b/f is the bound/free ratio, $\text{Ab}_T = \text{Ab} + \text{AgAb}$ the total concentration of antibody, $\text{Ag}_T = \text{Ag} + \text{AgAb}$ the total concentration of antigen, and B the concentration of bound antigen.

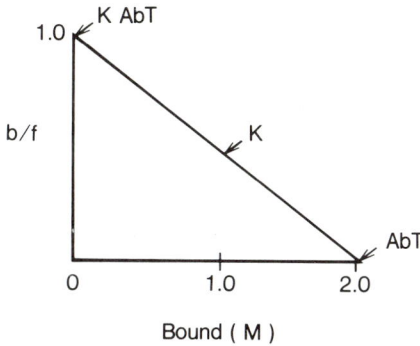

Figure 3. Scatchard plot.

The last equation indicates that there is a linear relationship between the bound-to-free ratio (b/f) and the concentration of bound antigen (B).

The graphic representation is known as a "Scatchard Plot." Two useful parameters can be determined from the Scatchard plot (Fig. 3): (**1**) the affinity constant (K) from the slope of the line and (**2**) the concentration of antibody binding sites (Ab_T) from the x intercept.

One can examine the effect of changing K and Ab_T on the nature of the Scatchard plot.

1. Increasing the antibody concentration shifts the curve to the right, while its slope remains unchanged (Fig. 4a).

2. If the affinity constant is increased, the curve pivots around the x intercept, moving to the right and steepening (Fig. 4b).

3. If the affinity constant is increased but the antibody concentration is decreased in proportion, the curve pivots around its y intercept, moving to the left and steepening (Fig. 4c).

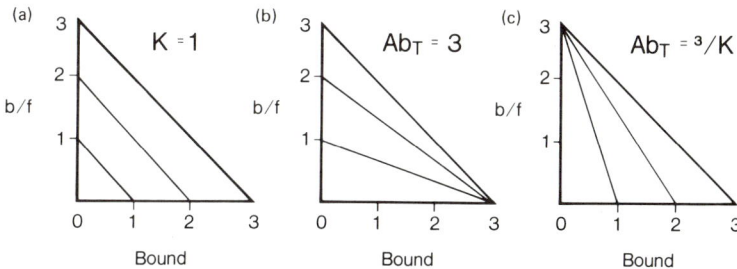

Figure 4. Scatchard plot: changing conditions.

C. Dose–Response Curve

The immunoassay reaction can be expressed with the total antigen and antibody concentrations in a dose–response curve.

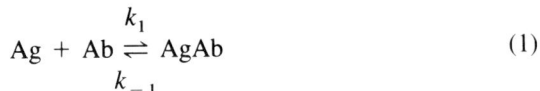

$$Ag + Ab \overset{k_1}{\underset{k_{-1}}{\rightleftharpoons}} AgAb \tag{1}$$

where Ag is the antigen, Ab the antibody, AgAb the antigen–antibody complex, k_1 the association rate constant, and k_{-1} the dissociation rate constant.

At equilibrium,

$$K = k_1/k_{-1} = (AgAb)/(Ag)(Ab) \tag{2}$$

The ratio of bound to free antigen (b/f) is

$$b/f = (AgAb)/(Ag) \tag{3}$$

and the components (Ag) and (Ab) are

$$(Ag) = (Ag_T) - (AgAb) \tag{4}$$

$$(Ab) = (Ab_T) - (AgAb) \tag{5}$$

where Ag_T is the total antigen concentration and Ab_T the total antibody concentration.

The ratio of bound to free antigen can be rearranged from Eqs. (3) and (4) to

$$b/f = (AgAb)/[(Ag_T) - (AgAb)]$$

Therefore,

$$(AbAb) = Ag_T(b/f)/[1 + (b/f)] \tag{6}$$

The dose–response equation can be obtained by combining Eqs. (2) and (3):

$$(b/f) = K(Ab) \tag{7}$$

and by substituting Eqs. (5) and (6) into Eq. (7):

$$(b/f) = K (Ab_T - \{Ag_T(b/f)/[1 + (b/f)]\})$$

Multiply by $1 + (b/f)$:

$$(b/f)(1 + b/f) - (1+b/f)KAb_T + (b/f)KAg_T = 0$$

$$(b/f)^2 + b/f - KAb_T - (b/f)KAb_T + (b/f)KAg_T = 0$$

$$(b/f)^2 + (b/f)(KAg_T - KAb_T + 1) - KAb_T = 0 \tag{8}$$

Equation (8) can be used to calculate b/f from each standard with known amount of total antigen Ag_T. A standard curve can be constructed by plotting b/f

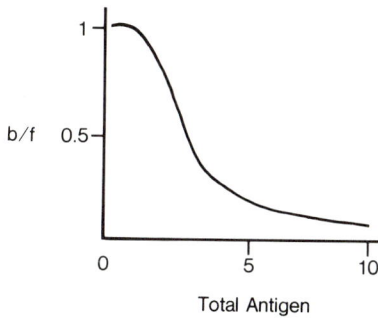

Figure 5. Typical RIA standard curve.

against Ag_T (Fig. 5). Therefore, an unknown sample for which b/f has been determined can be used to calculate the antigen concentration Ag_T. In a complex system involving multiple binding components, a simple graphic method can be used to determine each binding parameter (Rosenthal, 1967).

III. OPTIMIZATION OF IMMUNOASSAY

A. Reagent Components

The various types of immunoassay including enzyme immunoassay and fluorescence immunoassay will be discussed in more detail later in this chapter. The production of reagent components for immunoassay will be discussed in detail in Chapter 2. Here, I will only define the components.

1. Antigen: A substance that, when introduced into an animal, will induce the formation of antibodies. The antibody formed is found in serum and should react with the antigen used to induce its formation. A hapten is a substance, generally of low molecular weight, that by itself will not induce the formation of antibodies unless it is coupled to a carrier protein to form an antigen, for instance, steroid, thyroxine (T_4), and drugs.

2. Antibody: A serum protein belonging to the family called immunoglobulins (IgG, IgM, IgA, IgD, and IgE). Conventional immunization by injecting antigen into an animal stimulates the production of a heterogeneous population of antibodies that differ in their affinity and their specificity. Recently, the hybridoma technique has been used to produce monoclonal antibodies. The advantages of monoclonal antibodies are:

a. High specificity—a monoclonal antibody consists of a single determinant of the antigen.
b. Large quantity—there is an almost unlimited supply of antibodies.
c. Selectivity—there is a choice of characteristic antibodies.
3. Label: Labeled antigen or antibody, used to provide signal for quantitation. Common labels used in immunoassays are
   a. Radioactivity—the commonly used radioisotopes are ^{125}I, ^{57}Co for γ radiation, and ^3H and ^{14}C for β radiation.
   b. Enzyme—the enzyme labels include measurement of enzyme activity, enzyme inhibition, enzyme channeling to increase sensitivity, and enzymes involving luminescence.
   c. Fluorescence—fluorescence intensity, energy transfer, or polarization measurement may be used.

B. Optimization: Assay Sensitivity

In a competitive immunoassay, the dose–response curve is represented by Eq. (8):

$$(b/f)^2 + (b/f)(KAg_T - KAb_T + 1) - KAb_T = 0 \qquad (8)$$

where b/f is the ratio of bound to free antigen, K the affinity constant, Ag_T the total antigen concentration, and Ab_T the total antibody concentration.

Two approaches are used to optimize the assay sensitivity. Yalow and Benson (1970) defined sensitivity as the maximal slope of the standard curve independent of the experimental error. Ekins *et al.* (1970) defined sensitivity as the lower limit of detection, i.e., the least detectable dose.

1. Yalow and Benson's Model

In this model, the optimal conditions are $Ag_T = 0$ and $Ab_T = 0.5/K$. Therefore, Eq. (8) becomes

$$(b/f)^2 + (b/f)(0 - 0.5 + 1) - 0.5 = 0$$
$$(b/f)^2 + 0.5(b/f) - 0.5 = 0$$
$$(b/f + 1)(b/f - 0.5) = 0$$
$$b/f = -1; 0.5$$
$$b/\text{total} = 1/3, \text{ percent bound} = 33\%$$

The maximal slope is obtained with a initial percent bound of 33% when Ag_T approaches zero. This implies that maximal sensitivity can be obtained by using (a) a tracer with very high specific activity so that the initial antigen concentration approaches zero, (b) an antibody with a sufficiently large affinity constant at a concentration equal to $0.5/K$, and (c) an initial percent binding of 33%.

2. Ekin's Model

In this model, the optimal conditions are $Ag_T = 4/K$ and $Ab_T = 3/K$. Therefore, Eq. (8) becomes

$$(b/f)^2 + (b/f)(4 - 3 + 1) - 3 = 0$$

$$(b/f)^2 + 2(b/f) - 3 = 0$$

$$(b/f + 3)(b/f - 1) = 0$$

$$b/f = -3; 1$$

$$b/\text{total} = 1/2, \text{ percent bound} = 50\%$$

This implies that maximal sensitivity can be achieved with an initial percent binding of 50%. The lower limit of detection expressed as the least detectable dose (LDD) is inversely proportional to the square root of (1) the specific activity of the tracer, (2) the affinity constant, (3) the reaction volume, and (4) the counting time. Furthermore, this relationship is affected by the experimental error incurred in the measurement of bound and free antigens. An increase in the specific activity of the tracer will reduce the LDD (i.e., an increase in sensitivity), probably through a reduction in counting error. The affinity constant K and the experimental error are the limiting factors in achieving maximal sensitivity. Other factors such as reaction volume and counting time can provide limited compensation for the assay conditions (Ekins, 1981).

C. Factors Affecting Assay Conditions

Incubation of antigen and antibody allows the formation of an antigen–antibody complex. A number of factors affect the immunoassay reaction:

1. Temperature: Increased temperature generally increases the rate of the reaction between antigen and antibody. On the other hand, the affinity constant (K_a) generally decreases with increased temperature. Most naturally occurring binding proteins are much more sensitive to temperature changes. For example, the K_a for cortisol-binding globulin (transcortin) increased 20-fold as the temperature changed from 37 to 4°C (Chan and Slaunwhite, 1977), and K_a for thyroxine-binding globulin increased 3-fold from 37°C to room temperature. However, the affinity of T_4 for its antibody remained essentially unchanged. Therefore, higher sensitivity can be achieved at lower temperatures. Proteolysis and other adverse reactions, e.g., radioligand "damage," particularly with peptide hormone, occur at higher temperatures.

2. Incubation pH: The pH of the buffer is important in optimizing the binding reaction, particularly if the binding is pH-dependent. For example, pH 8.0 is optimal for the binding of cortisol to transcortin, the binding protein for cortisol in serum. In designing an RIA, one could take advantage of the temperature and

pH effect. For example, the binding of cortisol to transcortin is highly temperature-dependent, whereas the binding to antibody is not. By incubating at temperatures greater than 37°C and at pH 5, cortisol will be released from transcortin due to the low K_a at high temperature and low pH; however, its binding to antibody will be about the same. Therefore, the extraction of cortisol from its binder and the binding to antibody can be carried out in a single step, thereby eliminating the pretreatment of serum by heat denaturation.

3. Incubation time: Incubation of antigen and antibody to equilibrium requires a longer time, except for analytes with relatively high concentrations, e.g., thyroxine and cortisol. Sequential assay with the addition of unlabeled antigen before the labeled antigen can be used to increase the sensitivity and reduce the incubation time. This is particularly valuable for assays where the labeled antigen is sensitive to degradation. The exact incubation time becomes more critical with nonequilibrium techniques. For example, the time lag between pipetting the antibody to the first tube and the last tube may be 15–30 min, while they are centrifuged at the same time. The difference in the amount of antigen bound between tubes will be significant.

D. Immunometric Assay (IMA)

The optimal conditions for an immunometric assay are different from those for a competitive immunoassay. The sensitivity of IMA is essentially determined by the least detectable amount of the labeled antibody. Therefore, maximal sensitivity can be achieved with (1) high specific activity of the labeled antibody, (2) low nonspecific binding of the labeled antibody, (3) high affinity constant of the labeled antibody and antigen reaction, (4) small experimental errors in measuring the bound labeled antibody, and (5) large labeled antibody concentration (Ekins, 1981).

E. Separation Techniques

1. Heterogeneous Immunoassay

The method for the separation of free from bound antigen is based on the chemical or immunologic differences between free antigen and antigen–antibody complex. The differences utilized for separation include charge, size, solubility, immunologic determinants, and adsorption to solid materials. An ideal technique should be able to separate free and bound antigen completely and reproducibly without disturbing the equilibrium of the antigen–antibody reaction and without perturbing plasma components unique to the patient sample.

Separation methods will be discussed in more detail in Chapter 2. Some of the commonly used separation techniques include the following.

a. Double-antibody method: A second antibody from a different species of animal is used to precipitate the primary antigen–antibody complex. These complexes are then centrifuged out of solution.

b. Coated tube or plate: The reaction tube or microtitration plate is coated with primary antibody.

c. Solid phase: The antibody used is bonded to cellulose, Sephadex, or polystyrene beads.

d. Adsorption: Free antigen is adsorbed, e.g., with charcoal, while leaving the bound antigen in solution.

e. Solvent or salt: Antibody is precipitated and the bound fraction is counted, by adding a solvent or salt e.g., polyethylene glycol (PEG).

f. Column separation: Ion exchange or gel filtration may be used.

2. Homogeneous Immunoassay

There is no physical separation of bound and free components. In order to detect the changes occurring before and after antigen–antibody binding, one can take advantage of a number of parameters, including

a. Conformational change of enzyme
b. Inhibition of enzyme
c. Substrate-labeled fluorescence
d. Fluorescence energy transfer, protection, or polarization

IV. HETEROGENEOUS IMMUNOASSAY SYSTEMS

Heterogeneous immunoassay requires a separation step to separate free from bound antigen. Although the separation step is time-consuming and labor-intensive, it removes interfering substances from the patient serum before quantitation takes place. This also allows a larger sample size to be used, thereby increasing the sensitivity. Heterogeneous immunoassay is also more versatile. It can measure both small and large molecules. Homogeneous immunoassay such as the popular EMIT assay, on the other hand, measures only small molecules such as drugs.

These systems include the traditional radioimmunassay; immunometric assay with a radioactive label (IRMA); enzyme immunoassay, such as immunoassay with an enzyme label (IEMA) and enzyme-linked immunosorbent assay (ELISA); fluorescence immunoassay, such as particle concentration fluorescence immunoassay (PCFIA); and time-resolved fluoroimmunoassay. Comprehensive reviews of various immunoassays are given in books by Nakamura et al. (1980, 1984), Kaplan and Pesce (1981), and Boguslaski et al. (1984).

In this section I will highlight some nonisotopic immunoassay systems that are either common in clinical laboratories, interesting in principle, or unique in concept. I will not discuss the traditional RIA automation systems for the following reasons. Despite the availability of several different automation systems for RIA during the past 5–10 years, none of the systems has been widely used in clinical laboratories. Most systems require dedicated reagents from the same manufacturer. In my experience, the quality of reagents from the same manufacturer varies from analyte to analyte. Furthermore, most laboratories do not have sufficient patient samples to require the efficiency of a fully automated RIA system. With the exception of a few analytes such as T_4, cortisol, and those used in pregnancy tests, the majority of hormones are considered as ''low-volume'' tests.

A. Enzyme Immunoassay

Heterogeneous EIA using the traditional competitive approach has not been accepted in the clinical chemistry laboratory. It is obvious that this type of EIA is more labor-intensive than RIA, since it involves an extra step of adding substrate and incubation to measure product formation. However, its application with microtiter plates in microbiology and infectious diseases is widely accepted. EIA is an improvement over the classical microbiological assay, which is very time-consuming and imprecise.

Immunoenzymetric assay with the ''sandwich'' approach has been rather successful in replacing RIA. In order to form the sandwich, the antigen should have at least two distinct binding sites for antibodies. Therefore, this type of EIA can be used only to measure large analytes such as polypeptide hormones and enzymes. It is especially useful in the measurement of tumor markers, since most tumor markers are oncofetal proteins and enzymes. Manufacturers such as Abbott Laboratories and Hybritech, Inc., have many products using this approach. IEMA is rather specific for the analyte, particularly when combined with monoclonal antibodies (David *et al.*, 1981). For example, creatine kinase isoenzyme MB (CK-MB) has two subunits, M and B. By using two monoclonal antibodies, one directed against the M subunit and the other directed against the B subunit, one can eliminate interferences from CK-MM and CK-BB (Chan *et al.*, 1985). The other example is human chorionic gonadotropin, which has an α and a β subunit. Again, using two monoclonal antibodies, one directed against the α subunit and the other against the β subunit, one will measure only the hCG molecule. The IEMA can be performed as a simultaneous or sequential assay. In simultaneous IEMA (Fib. 2b), both labeled and unlabeled antibodies are incubated with the serum sample at the same time. The assay time is shorter and there are fewer pipetting steps. However, there is a potential for interferences from components in the serum sample. For example, a simultaneous IEMA for CK-MB using anti-M antibody coated on the bead and anti-B antibody labeled with enzyme may be subject to interference from samples containing high concentrations of CK-MM. The limited capacity of anti-M antibodies may be saturated with CK-MM, thereby preventing CK-MB from binding to the bead. On the other hand, a simultaneous IEMA for CK-MB using anti-B antibody coated on the bead and anti-M antibody labeled with enzyme could be subject to interference from high concentrations of CK-MM as well. The high CK-MM may bind to the enzyme-labeled anti-M antibodies and cause a severe reduction in the enzyme signal, for instance, a high-dose hook effect. A sequential assay (Fig. 2c) could minimize the interferences; however, the assay time becomes longer.

The Abbott system uses horseradish peroxidase conjugated to the antibody. The substrate, hydrogen peroxide and o-phenylenediamine · 2HCl, is converted by the enzyme to a colorimetric product and measured at 492 nm with a Quantum spectrophotometer.

The Hybritech reagent system, Tandem, uses the alkaline phosphatase conjugated to the antibody. The substrate, p-nitrophenyl phosphate, is converted by the enzyme to a colorimetric product and measured at 405 nm with a Photon spectrophotometer. In general, most Tandem calibration curves are linear, using two-point calibration.

B. Fluorescence Immunoassay

In fluorescence, a photon of an appropriate energy (excitation wavelength) excites the molecule from its ground state (S_0) to a higher electronic state (S_1). When the molecule returns to the ground state, energy is released as light emitted at a longer wavelength (emission wavelength). The difference between the excitation wavelength and the emission wavelength is the Stokes shift. A large Stokes shift in nanometers means that there is a large difference between the excitation and emission wavelengths. For example, fluorescein, a common fluorophore, has a small Stokes shift of 30 nm. It has a maximal absorption at 490 nm and emission at 520 nm. In contrast, a rare earth chelate such as europium has a large Stokes shift of 270 nm. It has a maximal absorption at 340 nm and an emission at 610 nm. The efficiency of the excited molecule in dissipating the energy by emission of light is termed the quantum yield and is defined as the ratio of the number of quanta emitted to the number of quanta absorbed.

In principle, a fluoroimmunoassay using fluorometry has an advantage over an enzyme immunoassay using colorimetry. In colorimetry, the light absorbed by a sample is related directly to the concentration of the absorbing molecule and is independent of the intensity. In fluorometry, the intensity of fluorescence emission is directly proportional to the intensity of the incident light. Therefore, the emission fluorescence (i.e., the signal of the system) can be increased by increasing the intensity of the incident light. Colorimetry involves two light beams of similar intensities, whereas in fluorometry the sample is detected against zero background (Smith *et al.*, 1981). Fluorometry is capable of detecting as little as 10^{-14} mol of a substance, whereas colorimetry can detect only 10^{-8} mol.

In practice, there are problems associated with fluorescence measurements. (1) Endogenous fluorophores, such as bilirubin and proteins, can increase the nonspecific background fluorescence and reduce the sensitivity of FIA. (2) Light scattering by high concentrations of protein, lipid, and other particles in serum will reduce the fluorescence signal. (3) The inner filter effect of hemoglobin and albumin will absorb part of the excitation or emission beam. (4) Quenching due to the nonspecific binding of albumin and the interaction with other specific quenching species may change the quantum yield of the fluorescence.

Therefore, the practical sensitivity of conventional fluoroimmunoassay in measuring substances in biological samples is much reduced. A number of steps can be taken to minimize these interferences, such as sample pretreatment with acid to precipitate proteins and other naturally fluorescent compounds, washing and separation of other interferences such as drugs, and careful selection of a filter so that the wavelengths of excitation and emission are far away from the interferences.

Heterogeneous fluoroimmunoassay requires a separation step to separate free from bound antigens. An important function of this step is the removal of endogenous fluorescent compounds and interfering substances from the sample prior to the detection step. This also allows large sample sizes to be used and improves sensitivity as well as specificity. Solid-phase FIA is a convenient approach either as competitive FIA or sandwich immunometric assay. An early application was in the quantitation of immunoglobulin. However, this simple technique has not gained much popularity in clinical chemistry. The principles and recent developments of fluoroimmunoassays and immunofluorometric assays have been reviewed (Hemmila, 1985).

Here I will discuss two recent FIA systems using different approaches to minimize some of the interferences. One uses particle concentration front-surface fluorescence, the other uses time-resolved fluorescence.

1. Particle Concentration Fluorescence Immunoassay

A fluorescence immunoassay system developed by Pandex Laboratories uses antibodies attached to solid-phase particles. The particles are concentrated on the well of a microtiter plate. The fluorescent signal of the plate is read by front-surface fluorometry (Jolley *et al.*, 1984).

The advantages of this system include (a) potential application to a wide range of analytes including both small and large molecules, (b) good sensitivity due to the fluorescent label, separation of interfering substances, and concentration of the signal, and (c) relatively short incubation time because the reaction takes place in a particle suspension.

In this system, antigen or antibody is bound to polystyrene latex (0.6–0.8 nm) particles. The particles are dispersed in solution, where the binding reaction takes place rapidly. Fluorescein-labeled antibodies are added and bound to the antigen or antibody, forming a sandwich on the particle. The reaction mixture is filtered through a 0.2-nm membrane at the bottom of the well. The trapped particles are washed. The particle-bound fluorescence is determined by front-surface fluorometry.

Preliminary applications include screening of antibodies as in hybridoma work and quantitation of immunoglobulin. Other potential applications of this technique include quantitation of large variety of analytes of interest, such as drugs and hormones.

2. Time-Resolved Fluoroimmunoassay

Another approach to FIA takes advantage of the differences in decay time between the fluorescent probe and the interfering substances (Soini and Kojola, 1983). Most biological materials have short-lived fluorescence (1–20 ns). Long-lived fluorophores (10–1000 μs) including rare earth metals such as Lanthanide chelates, europium, and terbium can be used as fluorescent probes. By using a time-resolved fluorometer, one can measure the long-lived fluorophore while rejecting the short-lived fluorescence of the interfering substances. In addition, the europium chelates have a relatively large quantum yield, a large Stokes shift with excitation at 340 nm and emission at 613 nm, negligible concentrations in biological samples, and are biochemically inert.

DELFIA, dissociation-enhanced lanthanide fluoroimmunoassay, is a time-resolved fluoroimmunoassay system manufactured by LKB-Wallac in Finland. The DELFIA technique involves an antibody labeled with a europium chelate (a lanthanide metal). The europium ion in this chelate is weakly fluorescent. With the addition of an enhancement solution, the europium ion is dissociated from its chelate and the fluorescence is intensified 10^6-fold. The DELFIA system uses microtitration strip wells in which either antibody (solid-phase sandwich DELFIA) or antigen (solid-phase competitive DELFIA) is attached to the wells. Each strip contains 12 wells. Eight strips are fitted into a holder to form a 96-well plate for pipetting. The Arcus fluorometer counts one strip at a time at the rate of 1 s per well.

The xenon flash lamp is activated about 1000 times (cycles) per second at a frequency of 1 kHz. Each cycle consists of an excitation at 340 nm, a delay time of 400 μs followed by a counting time of 400 μs at 613 nm, and a delay time of 200 μs before the next cycle starts. During the initial delay time, the interference from scattered light and short-lived (1–20 ns) fluorescence from biological materials can be virtually eliminated. This allows DELFIA to be very sensitive, on the order of 10^{-16} mol Eu^{3+} per cuvette. In addition, the lanthanide chelate has a very large Stokes shift of 273 μm, that is, the difference in wavelength between the excitation and emission spectral peaks. It has narrow emission maxima, which significantly reduces background fluorescence. The relatively large excitation region makes it possible to increase the specific activity of the lanthanide chelate label by increasing the excitation energy.

DELFIA, being a heterogeneous FIA, is versatile. Either competitive FIA or sandwich fluorometric assay can be used. Therefore, both small and large molecules can be measured. Diagnostic assay kits are available for hCG (Pettersson *et al.*, 1983), thyroid-stimulating hormone, luteinizing hormone, follicle-stimulating hormone, AFP, ferritin, HBsAg (Siitari *et al.*, 1983), cortisol, T_3, T_4, estradiol, testosterone, progesterone, digoxin, and rubella antibodies (Meurman *et al.*, 1982).

V. HOMOGENEOUS IMMUNOASSAY SYSTEMS

Homogeneous immunoassay eliminates the need for physical separation of bound from unbound antigen. This also allows a fully automated system to be developed for the clinical laboratory. Either the EIA or the FIA format is now frequently used. If the antigen is a small molecule, the bound antigen–antibody complex should be much larger than the antigen alone. Most homogeneous immunoassays take advantage of this difference in size or physical properties. Therefore, most homogeneous immunoassays can measure only analytes that are small molecules. The difference between the bound and unbound antigen defines the limit of fluorescence or spectrophotometric change and therefore the dynamic range of the assay.

Systems such as EMIT by Syva Corporation and TDx by Abbott Laboratories can measure only small molecules such as drugs and thyroxine. The sensitivity of these systems is adequate for most drug determinations; however, it is not sufficient for analytes such as T_3 and tricyclic antidepressants. Without separation of the serum sample, interferences can present problems. For example, the determination of digoxin on the TDx analyzer requires sample pretreatment to minimize interferences.

A. Enzyme Immunoassay System

In contrast to heterogeneous EIA, where the enzyme label plays a passive role in the immunoassay reaction, the enzyme in homogeneous EIA plays a much more active role. The change of signal is dependent on enzyme inhibition, activation, or conformational changes. Understanding of the enzymology is much more critical in homogeneous FIA. For many years, drug assays for therapeutic monitoring were performed by chromatographic techniques. Nonisotopic immunoassays now dominate therapeutic drug monitoring in most clinical laboratories. The most widely used homogeneous enzyme immunoassay

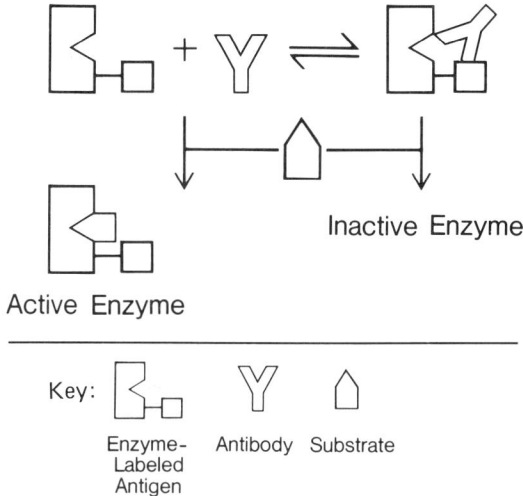

Active Enzyme

Inactive Enzyme

Key:

Enzyme-   Antibody Substrate
Labeled
Antigen

Figure 6. Principle of EMIT assay.

is the EMIT technique developed by Syva. The majority of EMIT assays are for therapeutic drug monitoring and detection of drug abuse. The EMIT assay can be performed with a simple spectrophotometer or an automated chemistry analyzer. Centrifugal analyzers such as Encore (Baker), Monarch (Instrumentation Laboratory), and Cobas-Bio and MIRA (Roche Diagnostics) have been adapted to perform EMIT assays. The combined system allows micro sample volume, small reagent usage, and fully automated testing for EMIT assays.

EMIT assays use an enzyme label such as glucose-6-phosphate dehydrogenase (G6PDH), malate dehydrogenase (MDH), or lysozyme. The enzyme label is coupled to a drug derivative. The unbound form of the enzyme-labeled drug derivative is active in solution and can act on the substrate to form a product. On binding to an antibody, the activity of the enzyme decreases as a result of inhibition or conformational change (Fig. 6). This difference in enzyme activity between bound and free drug derivative is measured by the NADH concentration at 340 nm in a spectrophotometer. A long list of TDM drugs and drugs of abuse can be measured by this technique (Crowl *et al.*, 1980).

B. Fluorescence Immunoassay System

There are a number of approaches to homogeneous fluorescence immunoassay, including fluorescence polarization immunoassay (FPIA), substrate-labeled fluoroimmunoassay (SLFIA), fluorescence enhancement immunoassay, indirect quenching fluoroimmunoassay, fluorescence excitation transfer immunoassay (FETIA), and fluorescence protection immunoassay (FPIA) (Hemmila,

1985). Only the first two approaches, FPIA and SLFIA, have gained much commercial success. Here, I will discuss these two assay systems.

1. Substrate-Labeled Fluoroimmunoassay

SLFIA falls in the category of release fluoroimmunoassay. The principle is based on the presence of a hydrolyzable bond between an antigen and a fluorescent probe. Most common releasable quenching bonds are ester and glycoside bonds in the umbelliferone derivative. The probe is not fluorescent in this complex form. However, it can be converted to a fluorescent product by an enzyme.

The TDA system developed by Ames Division of Miles Laboratories is a competitive fluoroimmunoassay based on the SLFIA principle. In this system, the substrate-labeled antigen bound to antibody cannot react with the enzyme; however, the unbound substrate-labeled antigen can be converted to a fluorescent product (Fig. 7). The fluorogenic substrate, β-galactosylumibelliferone, is weakly fluorescent. It has excitation and emission maxima at 350 and 400 nm, respectively. After the enzymatic hydrolysis, the maxima shift to 400 and 450 nm. The fluorescence intensity also increases 10- to 15-fold (Boguslaski *et al.*, 1980). The fluorescence can be measured by a simple fluorometer or by Optimate, an automated fluorometer from Ames Division of Miles Laboratories. One advantage of this system is its ability to measure both small and large molecules including drugs and proteins. An extensive list of TDM assays is available. Filter paper disks or strips containing all the necessary reagents are also available. With

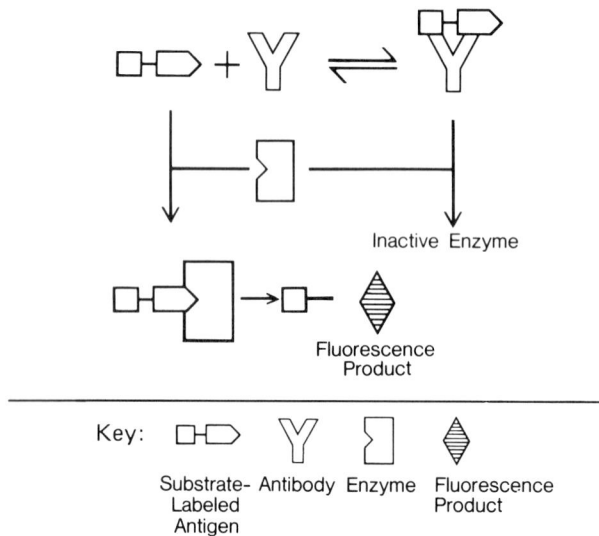

Figure 7. Principle of substrate-labeled fluoroimmunoassay.

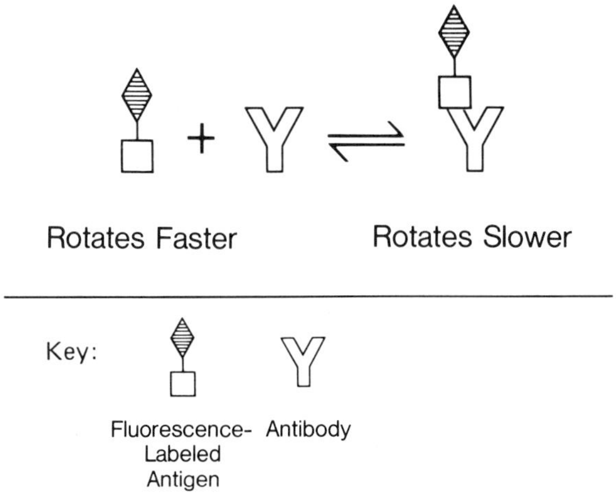

Rotates Faster   Rotates Slower

Key:

Fluorescence- Antibody
Labeled
Antigen

Figure 8. Principle of fluorescence polarization immunoassay.

the addition of patient sample, the fluorescent signal can be measured by a desktop fluorometer.

2. Fluorescence Polarization Immunoassay

When a fluorescent molecule is excited with polarized light, the resulting emission depends on the rotational property of the molecule. A small molecule, such as a fluorescent labeled antigen, rotates faster in solution than a large molecule, such as an antigen–antibody complex (Fig. 8). When polarized light excites the small molecule, which is rotating faster, the polarization signals decrease more than those of the large molecule. In a competitive FPIA, the added unlabeled antigen competes with the fluorescent labeled antigen for the antibody binding sites. With increasing concentration of unlabeled antigen, more fluorescent labeled antigen becomes unbound. Therefore, the fluorescence polarization signal decreases (Dandliker *et al.*, 1980). Abbott Laboratories developed an automated TDx system based on the FPIA principle. An extensive list of assays of drugs and hormones is available. The major advantage of the TDx reagent is the stability of its calibration curve for at least 4 weeks. The automated TDx assay is also very rapid. Recently, Roche Diagnostics also developed FPIA for drug determination on its chemistry analyzer, the Cobas system.

REFERENCES

Adams, R. F., and Vandemark, F. L. (1976). Simultaneous high-pressure liquid-chromatographic determination of some anticonvulsants in serum. *Clin. Chem.* **22,** 25–31.

Boguslaski, R. C., Li, T. M., Benovic, J. L., Ngo, T. T., Burd, J. F., and Carrice, R. C. (1980). Substrate labeled homogeneous fluorescent immunoassays for haptens and proteins. In "Immunoassays: Clinical Laboratory Techniques for the 1980's" (R. M. Nakamura, W. R. Dito, and E. S. Tucker III, eds.), pp. 45–64. Alan R. Liss, New York.

Boguslaski, R. C., Maggio, E. T., and Nakamura, R. M. (1984). "Clinical Immunochemistry: Principles of Methods and Application." Little, Brown, Boston.

Campfield, L. A. (1983). Mathematical analysis of competitive protein binding assays. In "Principles of Competitive Protein-Binding Assays" (W. Odell and P. Franchimont, eds.), 2nd ed., pp. 125–148. John Wiley & Sons, New York.

Chan, D. W., and Slaunwhite, W. R. (1977). The chemistry of human transcortin. II. The effects of pH, urea, salt and temperature on the binding of cortisol and progesterone. *Arch. Biochem. Biophys.* **182,** 437–442.

Chan, D. W., Taylor, E., Frye, R., and Blitzer, R.-L. (1985). Immunoenzymetric assay for creatine kinase MB with subunit-specific monoclonal antibodies compared with an immunochemical method and electrophoresis. *Clin. Chem.* **31,** 405–569.

Chan, D. W., Kelsten, M., Rock, R., and Bruzek, D. (1986). Evaluation of a monoclonal immunoenzymometric assay for alpha-fetoprotein. *Clin Chem.* **32,** 1318–1322.

Crowl, C. P., Gibbons, I., and Schneider, R. S. (1980). Recent advances in homogeneous enzyme immunoassays for haptens and proteins. In "Immunoassays: Clinical Laboratory Techniques for the 1980's" (R. M. Nakamura, W. R. Dito, and E. S. Tucker III, eds.), pp. 89–126. Alan R. Liss, New York.

Dandliker, W. B., Hsu, M.-L., and Vanderlaan, W. P. (1980). Fluorescence polarization immuno/receptor assays. In "Immunoassays: Clinical Laboratory Techniques for the 1980's" (R. M. Nakamura, W. R. Dito, and E. S. Tucker III, eds.), pp. 65–88. Alan R. Liss, New York.

David, G. S., Wang, R., Bartholomew, R., Sevier, E. D., Adams, T., and Greene, H. E. (1981). The hybridoma—an immunochemical laser. *Clin. Chem.* **27,** 1580–1585.

Ekins, R. (1981). Toward immunoassays of greater sensitivity, specificity and speed: an overview. In "Monoclonal Antibodies and Developments in Immunoassay" (A. Albertini and R. Ekins, eds.), pp. 3–21. Elsevier/North-Holland Biomedical Press, New York.

Ekins, R. P., Newman, G. B., and O'Riordan, J. L. H. (1970). Saturation assays. In "Statistics in Endocrinology" (J. W. McArthur and J. Colton, eds.), pp. 345–378. MIT Press, Cambridge, Massachusetts.

Hemmila, I. (1985). Fluoroimmunoassays and immunofluorometric assays. *Clin. Chem.* **31,** 359–370.

Jolley, M. E., Wang, E. H., Ekenber, S. J., Zuelke, M. S., and Kelso, D. M. (1984). Particle concentration fluorescence immunoassay (PCFIA): a new, rapid immunoassay technique with high sensitivity. *J. Immunol. Methods* **67,** 21–35.

Kabra, P. M., Koo, H. Y., and Marton, L. J. (1978). Simultaneous liquid-chromatographic determination of 12 common sedatives and hypnotics in serum. *Clin. Chem.* **24,** 657–662.

Kaplan, L. A., and Pesce, A. J. (1981). In "Nonisotopic Alternatives to Radioimmunoassay: Principle and Applications." Marcel Dekker, New York.

Least, C. J., Johnson, G. F., and Solomon, H. M. (1975). Therapeutic monitoring of anticonvulsant drugs: gas-chromatographic simultaneous determination of primidone, phenyethylmalonamide, carbamazepine, and diphenylhydantoin. *Clin. Chem.* **21,** 1658–1662.

Meurman, O. H., Hemmila, I. A., Lovgren, T., and Halonen, P. E. (1982). Time-resolved fluoroimmunoassay: a new test for rubella antibodies. *J. Clin. Microbiol.* **16,** 920–925.

Nakamura, R. M., Dito, W. R., and Tucker, E. S., III (1980). Immunoassay: Clinical Laboratory Techniques for the 1980's. Alan R. Liss, New York.

Nakamura, R. M., Dito, W. R., and Tucker, E. S., III (1984). In "Clinical Laboratory Assays: New Technology and Future Directions." Masson, New York.

Pettersson, K., Siitari, H., Hemmila, I., Soini, E., Lorgren, T., Hanninen, V., Tanner, P., and Stenman, U.-H. (1983). Time-resolved fluoroimmunoassay of human choriogonadotropin. *Clin. Chem.* **29,** 60–64.

Rosenthal, H. E. (1967). A graphic method for the determination and presentation of binding parameters in a complex system. *Anal. Biochem.* **20,** 525–532.

Saxena, B. B., Hasan, S. H., Haour, F., and Schmidt-Gollwitzer, M. (1974). Radioreceptor assay of human chorionic gonadotropin: detection of early pregnancy. *Science* **184,** 793–795.

Scatchard, G. (1949). The attractions of proteins for small molecules and ions. *Ann. N.Y. Acad. Sci.* **51,** 660–672.

Siitari, H., Hemmila, I., Soini, E., and Lorgren, T. (1983). Detection of hepatitis B surface antigen using time-resolved fluoroimmunoassay. *Nature (London)* **301,** 258–260.

Smith, D. S., Al-Hakiem, M. H., and Laudon, J. (1981). A review of fluoroimmunoassay and immunofluorometric assay. *Ann. Clin. Biochem.* **18,** 253–274.

Soini, E., and Kojola, H. (1983). Time resolved fluorometer of lanthanide chelates—a new generation of nonisotopic immunoassays. *Clin. Chem.* **29,** 65–68.

Yalow, R. S., and Benson, S. A. (1970). Proceedings of symposium on "in vitro" procedures with radioisotopes in clinical medicine and research, pp. 455–470. Vienna, IAFA, SM-124-106.

Chapter 2

Production of Immunoassay Reagents

Robert G. Hamilton

Rheumatology and Clinical
Immunogenetics Division
Department of Internal Medicine
University of Texas School of Medicine
Houston, Texas 77025

I. INTRODUCTION

Advances in biochemistry, immunology, and molecular biology continue to provide laboratorians with more pure and well-characterized immunoassay reagents. The preparation of these reagents, however, is generally beyond the technical capability of most clinical immunoassay laboratories. The objective of this chapter is to review and provide recent references for commonly employed reagents in five major categories: receptors or binders, unlabeled ligands–calibrators, labeled ligands and labeled binders, separation reagents, and assay buffers. This chapter should be considered an overview of methods for educational purposes rather than a detailed collection of immunochemical facts and protocols sufficient for the complete preparation of the immunoassay reagents. Its intent is to provide a summary of significant achievements in the field of immunoassay reagent preparation while at the same time providing a reference compendium of widely used techniques. The discussion in this chapter will assume an understanding of the principles of competitive and noncompetitive, homogeneous and heterogeneous immunoassay designs presented in Chapter 1.

II. RECEPTORS OR BINDERS

The receptor or binder is the immunoassay reagent which restricts the movement of labeled and unlabeled ligands in solution to the degree that it has an

Table I. Overview of Ligand Assay Binding Reagents

Properties	Antisera	Tissue receptor	Carrier proteins
General use	Widest	Limited	Limited
Affinity	Potentially the highest	Very high	High
(in liters/mole)	(10^{10}–10^{12})	(10^9–10^{11})	(10^8)
Specificity	Variable	Very high	High
Preparation time	Months	Hours	Minutes
Method	Animal (polyclonal) Cells (monoclonal)	Cell fractionation	Serum dilution
Reproducibility	Variable (polyclonal) Consistent (monoclonal)	Consistent	Consistent
Long-term storage	Very stable	Unstable	Very stable

affinity or attractive force for the ligand that causes it to enter into and remain in chemical combination. The properties of the receptor define the nature (magnitude) of the competitive and noncompetitive binding reactions with labeled and unlabeled ligands and binders within constraints of dynamic equilibrium, the law of mass action, the isotope dilution principle, and Le Chatelier's principle as described in exhaustive detail by multiple authors (Berson and Yalow, 1973; Ekins, 1974; Thorell and Larson, 1978; Chard, 1983; Odell and Daughaday, 1983) and summarized in Chapter 1.

A. Receptor Types

Historically, polyclonal human antibodies (Berson and Yalow, 1959) and plasma transport proteins such as thyroxine-binding globulin (Ekins, 1960) and transcortin (Murphy *et al.*, 1963) were among the earliest receptors employed in ligand binding assays. The use of rabbit uterine cytosol as a receptor for plasma estradiol (E_2) provided early evidence that tissue receptors could be used successfully to measure ligands (Korenman, 1968). The most widely used of the receptors, however, have been polyclonal antibody and more recently monoclonal antibody due to their versatility in terms of specificity, availability, and stability. Table I summarizes general properties of the three major classes of binders (antisera, tissue receptors, and serum carrier proteins) that are widely used in ligand binding assays.

B. Polyclonal Antibody Production

Antibody is a protein which is formed as part of an immune response to a foreign substance (immunogen), combines specifically with the immunogen, and, to a variable extent, can cross-react with substances of similar structure. There is no perfect recipe for the preparation of polyclonal antibodies in rabbits, goats, and sheep. General principles governing the selection of the animal for immunization, preparation of the immunogen, use of adjuvants, calculation of the amount of immunogen to be injected, selection of the route of injection and the injection schedules, and collection and storage of antisera are discussed in detail by Chase (1967), Harboe and Ingild (1975), and Franchimont *et al.* (1983). Once produced in the serum of the animal, antibody can be collected and readily characterized by immunoprecipitation (Kabat, 1976) and radioimmunoassay (Hamilton, 1980; Parratt *et al.*, 1982). Site-specific antibodies can be isolated from the serum by first isolating the immunoglobulin fraction with ion-exchange resin chromatography, affinity purifying or extracting specific antibody from the total IgG fraction with antigen covalently coupled to cyanogen bromide–activated agarose, and finally eluting bound antibodies with chaotropic agents such as glycine-HCl buffer, pH 2.4 (Table II).

Table II. Selected Immunoassay Buffer Systems[a]

---

1. Borate buffer, pH 7.4, 0.2 M
   Borate solution: 9.54 g disodium tetraborate ($Na_2B_4O \cdot 10H_2O$ in 250 ml distilled water.
   Boric acid: 24.73 g in 4 liters of distilled water.
   Add approximately 115 ml borate solution to 4 liters of boric acid solution until pH reaches 7.4.
2. Borate-buffered saline, pH 8.3–8.5, 0.1 M
   Add boric acid (6.18 g/liter) to a 1000-liter flask.
   Add sodium tetraborate (borax) (9.54 g/liter) and sodium chloride (4.38 g/liter).
   Reconstitute to 1000 ml with distilled water.
3. Carbonate buffer, pH 9.6, 0.05 M
   Dissolve sodium carbonate (Na_2CO_3, 1.59 g/liter) and sodium hydrogen carbonate ($NaHCO_3$, 2.93 g/liter) to a final volume of 1000 ml with distilled water.
4. Citrate buffer (pH 3.0–7.0), 0.1 M
   Prepare 0.1 M citric acid ($C_6H_8O_7 \cdot 1H_2O$, 21.01 g/liter).
   Prepare 0.1 M disodium hydrogen phosphate ($Na_2HPO_4 \cdot 2H_2O$, 35.6 g/liter)
   For pH 5.0: approximately 50 : 50 mixture citric to phosphate
   For pH < 5.0: titrate pH of citric acid with phosphate.
   For pH > 5.0: titrate pH of phosphate with citric acid.
5. Glycine–hydrochloric acid buffer, pH 2.5 or 2.8, 0.1 M (for acid elution of antibodies from an immunosorbent column)
   Titrate pH of 500 ml of 0.2 M glycine (15.01 g/liter) to 2.5–2.8 with 0.2 M hydrochloric acid. Make up to 1 liter.
6. Phosphate-buffered saline (PBS), pH 7.2, 0.15 M
   Dissolve sodium chloride (8.00 g/liter), potassium chloride (0.20 g/liter), disodium hydrogen phosphate (Na_2HPO_4) (1.15 g/liter = 0.008 M), potassium dihydrogen phosphate (0.20 g/liter) into a final volume of 1 liter of distilled water.
7. Veronal-buffered saline (5× concentrate)
   Add sodium chloride (85 g), sodium barbitone (3.75 g), and barbitone (5.75 g) to distilled water to make a final volume of 2 liters. Store as the 5× concentrate because it is more stable and dilute 1 : 5 just before use.

---

[a]All solutions must be made with deionized double or triple distilled water.

The more successful regimens of immunization have several factors in common. The immunogen needs to be carefully prepared prior to use in immunization. This involves its purification and the coupling of smaller molecules (haptens; MW typically <1000) to larger proteins (carriers) (Abraham and Grover, 1971). Antigen is frequently emulsified with an adjuvant composed of mineral oil with microbacteria (complete form) or without microbacteria (incomplete form) to heighten the animal's immune response following immunization (Freund and Thomson, 1948).

C. Monoclonal Antibody Production

A technique that has revolutionized antibody production is the cell hybridization method first described by Kohler and Milstein (1975). In this procedure, antibody-secreting spleen cells are fused with "immortal" myeloma cells to produce a hybridoma cell line. Unlimited quantities of antibodies with restricted specificity can be prepared by this method, which eliminates concern over the use of large quantities of antibody in the sensitive immunoradiometric assay (IRMA) that employs a sandwich of labeled and solid-phase antibodies to detect ligands (Hales and Woodhead, 1980).

An schematic of the monoclonal antibody hybridoma technique is depicted in Fig. 1. The method involves the immunization of mice with antigen followed weeks later with a booster of the same antigen. Days after the booster, the spleen is removed and mouse lymphocytes (approximately 10^8 cells) are fused in the presence of polyethylene glycol with cultured mouse myeloma cells (2×10^7) that are deficient in the enzyme hypoxanthine-guanine ribosyltransferase (HAT). The fused cells (heterokaryons) are cultured in a medium containing HAT that prevents growth of the myeloma cells. The mouse lymphocytes normally die after a week, leaving only the heterokaryon colonies that possess the combined traits of the lymphocytes and myeloma cells. These cultures are called hybridomas. They are cloned and the daughter cells are screened for the production of specific antibody by microtiter plate enzyme or radioimmunoassay methods. A clone of cells that secretes a specific antibody of interest is further cloned, mass-produced in ascites, and frozen away for future use. Quality control of murine monoclonal antibodies is commonly performed using a combination of assays. Microtiter plate-based immunoassays are useful in quantifying the amount and monitoring the degree of specificity of antibody in culture medium and ascites. Isoelectric focusing affinity immunoblot analysis is a new technique for long-term monitoring of monoclonal antibody production using the antibody's unique isoelectric point fingerprint as a marker of consistency (Hamilton et al., 1987). Details of methods for production, screening, and testing of monoclonal antibodies are presented in the textbook by Goding (1983).

Monoclonal antibodies have been used widely in the noncompetitive IRMA configuration to detect molecules with a wide spectrum of sizes as exemplified

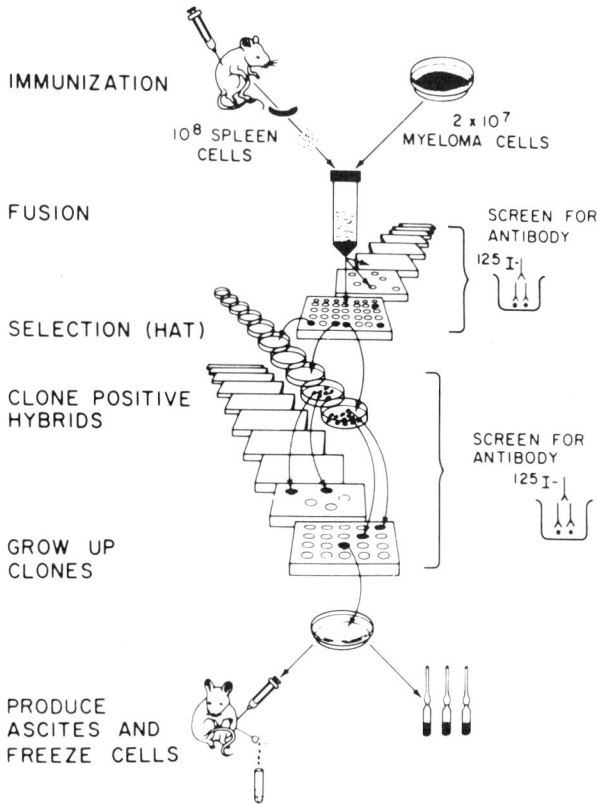

Figure 1. Hybridoma technique for the production of monoclonal antibody. Spleen cells from an immunized mouse are fused with mouse myeloma cells in the presence of polyethylene glycol. The hybrids formed survive a process of selection in HAT growth medium and clones producing the specific antibody of interest are isolated after careful screening using a immunometric assay. Once isolated, the clones of interest are cultured, mass-produced in ascites, and frozen for future use. Spleen and myeloma cells from other specific have also been used with varying degrees of success. (Reproduced with permission from Hamilton and Waud, 1982.)

by human interferon (Secher, 1981), carcinoembryonic antigen (Shively, 1984), and human IgE (David *et al.,* 1981). Selection of an ideal pair of monoclonal antibodies that recognize different determinants which are sterically distinct on the ligand molecule has permitted rapid simultaneous addition of labeled and solid-phase antibody to the assay reaction mixture without loss of assay sensitivity. Sensitivity of a two-site labeled-antibody assay employing two specifities of monoclonal antibody can be further manipulated by selecting the antibody clone with the best affinity for the desired working range of the assay. This "immunoengineering" has ushered in a new era in immunoassay receptor production.

D. Tissue Receptors

Despite the limited use of tissue receptors in clinical ligand binding assays, these binders possess the distinct advantages of very high affinity, specificity for biologically active ligands, and short preparation time. The radioreceptor assay provides a unique amalgamation of the sensitivity of immunoassay with the specificity of bioassays that measure biologically relevant rather than strictly immunoreactive analytes. The importance of detecting biologically active ligands has been emphasized by Belcher (1984), who overviews the many types of receptors that have been identified and used as binders, and by Saxena (1981), who discusses a specific case, the relative merits of pregnancy tests that use tissue receptors instead of antibody for the measurement of β human chorionic gonadotropin in serum.

Monoclonal antibodies have been employed in the purification and characterization of many cell surface receptors (Fraser and Lindstrom, 1984). Cell receptors that have been isolated by using solid-phase monoclonal antibodies and/or studied with labeled monoclonal antibody probes include the red cell β-adrenergic receptor (Fraser and Venter, 1982), calf uterus estrogen receptor (Greene *et al.*, 1980), human placental insulin receptor (Kull *et al.*, 1982), adrenal cortex low-density lipoprotein receptor (Beisiegel *et al.*, 1981), nicotinic acetylcholine receptor (Lindstrom *et al.*, 1985), thyrotropin receptors (Yavin *et al.*, 1981), and transferrin receptor human hematopoietic cells (Trowbridge and Lopez, 1982). The isolation of receptors from membranes of cells can be facilitated by using biotinylated monoclonal antibodies followed by extraction from the fluid phase with solid-phase streptavidin (see avidin–biotin in Sec. IV,B) (Updyke and Nicolson, 1984). Human autoantibodies can also be used to extract receptors and probe receptor structure and function (Harrison, 1984).

E. Serum Binding Proteins

Transport proteins represent a third group of binders that are employed in ligand assays for low-molecular-weight hormones and vitamins. The most widely used proteins in this group are thyroxine-binding globulin (TBG), transcortin, intrinsic factor (the gastric mucosa vitamin B_{12} transport protein), and sex hormone-binding globulin. While these proteins were commonly used as binders in early assays, they have to a large extent been replaced by specific antibodies.

F. Assay Properties Influenced by Receptor Quality

The ligand binding assay's sensitivity (minimal dose detectable with good precision) is one assay parameter directly influenced by the avidity or strength with which a receptor binds to its ligand. It is generally not necessary to calculate the avidity of the antibody, but it is useful to define the actual sensitivity (smallest quantity detectable with good precision) under test assay conditions. The affinity constant (K_a) is a good parameter for comparing the binding properties of multiple antisera, and its measurement by Scatchard analysis is discussed in Chapter 3.

The second assay performance parameter affected by the receptor quality is specificity or the ability to detect a single substance in a heterogeneous mixture. Analysis of increasing quantities of potentially cross-reacting substances in the assay as test samples will provide information on the degree of specificity afforded by the receptor. All unrelated and chemically related compounds that may occur in the biological specimen should be tested in a cross-reactivity study as described in Chapter 3.

III. UNLABELED LIGANDS—CALIBRATORS

A ligand is the substance (analyte) which is bound by receptor. A calibration standard may be defined as a solution containing a matrix (generally protein) and a defined quantity of the test analyte of interest. The calibrator provides a measurable degree of binding or displacement for a fixed, known quantity of ligand. Pure chemicals are usually measured in terms of mass concentration (grams per liter) or substance concentration (moles per liter). Biologically active substances are assayed in terms of biological standards and units of activity. When the exact concentration in weight per volume units or the biological activity units are not known, it is common to assign arbitrary units such as international units. Biological standards and reference materials are provided by several agencies (World Health Organization, American National Pituitary Agency, National Institute for Biological Standards and Control) and defined by their lot, units of biological activity and/or weight per volume, and a description of the carrier matrix which prevents loss on the ampule (protein, lactose, salts) (Hamilton and Adkinson, 1987).

The general requirements for the standard or calibrator are that it represent the native molecule to be quantitated in terms of purity and homogeneity, be stable over its indicated shelf life, be supplied in a usable protein matrix which emulates test specimens (serum, plasma, urine) (Kubasik and Sine, 1976), and be defined in terms of biological (activity), immunological (degree of immunoreactivity), and/or chemical (weight per volume) units (Duncan et al., 1984). A recent evaluation of a reference serum for human antibodies to DNA demonstrates the problems encountered when a new standard is being analyzed in multiple centers and results in different assays are generated in noncompatible units (Berne et al., 1984).

Stability is a problem for some plasma polypeptide hormones such as angiotensins I and II, glucagon, parathyroid hormone, and bradykinin. These ligands are highly susceptible to degradation by proteolytic enzymes in the blood and can be unstable when isolated. To minimize breakdown by oxidants and/or proteolytic enzymes in both reference and test specimens, chelating agents and/or proteinase inhibitors such as aprotinin (Trasylol) can be included in assay buffers (Eisentraut *et al.*, 1968). In some cases, test ligands are isolated prior to assay, which reduces nonspecific binding and interference from cross-reacting ligands. Extraction or preisolation does reduce proteolytic enzyme degradation, but it increases the work and the turnaround time and creates a need for recovery studies to monitor possible losses during isolation.

IV. LABELED LIGANDS AND RECEPTORS

Multiple isotopic and nonisotopic labels have been used throughout the years as tracers in immunoassays. Historically, the radiolabel provided a tracer which was simple to measure, unaffected by its chemical environment, and sufficiently small that it did not alter binding kinetics in the reaction mixture. Criticism of the use of radiolabels has focused on their relatively short half-life, the relatively long counting times required to achieve good statistical accuracy (10,000 counts for 1% variation), their limited shelf life, the expense of disposal, and concern over general laboratory safety (Maggio, 1980). Despite the continual prediction of doom for isotopic labels, they continue to be widely used in both clinical and research laboratories. Their continued use stems in part from the ease of reagent preparation and optimization, a history of good reproducible performance, and the wide availability of γ-counting equipment. Table III summarizes the most widely employed isotopic and nonisotopic labels in the immunoassay laboratory.

A. Isotopic Labels

Iodine-125 is the most widely used isotopic marker for labeled ligands and binders, primarily because of the readily available radioiodination methods. Most procedures which have been reported include the chloramine-T, lactoperoxidase, iodogen, and Bolton–Hunter methods. The fundamental principle governing the first three methods is the oxidation of the iodide (-1 valence) shipped as NaI (pH 10–11) to a $+1$ valence form in which one or two molecules bind to the benzene ring of tyrosine or histamine residues in proteins. The reaction is stopped by reducing all unreacted molecules to a -1 valence or separating unbound from bound radioiodine on a molecular sieve gel column.

In the chloramine-T method, *N*-chloro-*p*-toluenesulfonamide oxidizes the iodide while *meta*-bisulfite reduces the remaining unreacted radioiodine (Greenwood *et al.*, 1963). The lactoperoxidase procedure uses a more gradual oxidation of the iodide in the presence of peroxide, and the reaction is stopped by separat-

Table III. Labels Employed in Immunoassays

Isotopic labels

Isotope	Half-life	Decay type	Energy	Specific activity (mCi/µg)
^{125}I	60.2 d	Electron capture	28 and 35 keV x rays	17.3
^{35}S	87.9 d	Beta decay	167 keV beta	—
^{14}C	5760 yr	Beta decay	158 keV beta	0.0044
^{3}H	12.3 yr	Beta decay	18 keV beta	9.7

Nonisotopic Labels

Enzymes	Luminescence
Alkaline phosphatase	Luminol
Horseradish peroxidase	Acridium esters
β-D-Galactosidase	Electronic spin resonance
Penicillinase	Nitroxide radical
Urease	2,4-Dinitrophenyl
Fluorescence	Other
Fluorescein isothiocyanate	T₄ bacteriophage that kills *Escherichia coli*
Rhodamine	
Galactosylumbelliferone	
Tetramethylrhodamine isothiocyanate	

ing the enzyme from the iodinated material by either column chromatography or solid-phase separation (Thorell and Johansson, 1971). These two methods have been compared by many with the conclusion that they produce comparable results; chloramine-T produces high specific activity iodinated ligands, some of which are damaged, while lactoperoxidase produces a less damaged, more immunoreactive population of iodinated molecules (Ghanem *et al.*, 1982). More recently, iodogen (1,3,4,6-tetrachloro-3*a*,6*a*-diphenylglycouril), which performs a mild oxidation of iodide, has been introduced (Fraker and Speck, 1978). In a manner similar to lactoperoxidase, iodogen produces a mildly iodinated molecule that exhibits minimal damage and high immunoreactivity at the expense of very high specific activities (Lee and Griffiths, 1984).

For molecules that have no tyrosines or have tyrosines in binding regions of the molecule, the Bolton–Hunter reagent (an iodinated *p*-hydroxyphenylpropionic acid, *N*-hydroxysuccinimide ester) has been used successfully. It acylates terminal or lysine amino groups with an iodinated residue and thus incorporates radioiodine into proteins that do not have accessible tyrosines (Bolton and Hunter, 1973). Diazotized sulfanilic acid (^{35}S) and diazotized iodosulfanilic acid (^{125}I) are similar reagents used for radiolabeling the histidines and tyrosines of cell membrane surface proteins (Carraway, 1975). These acids cannot enter into the interior of cells, and thus they label only exposed membrane molecules. One

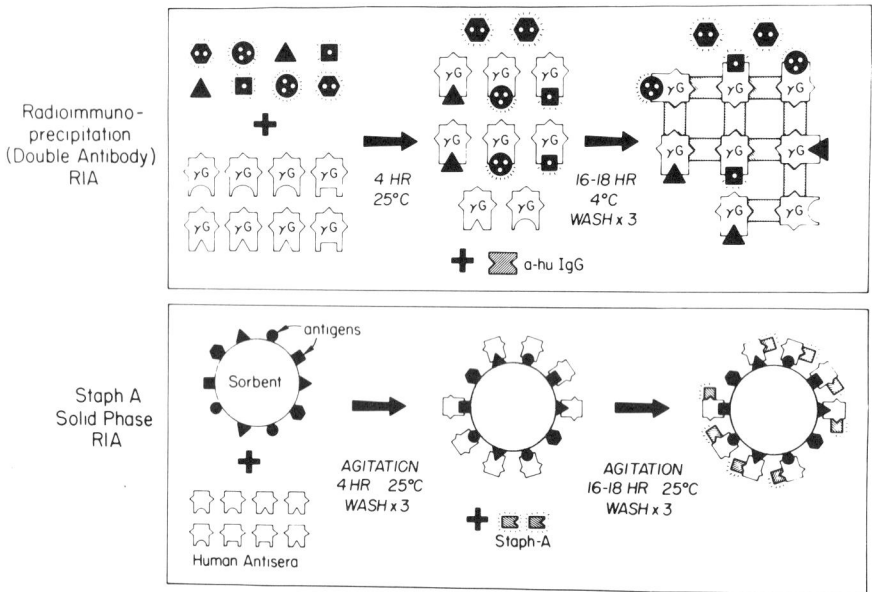

Figure 2. Schematic diagram illustrating the principles of quantitation of antigen-specific IgG antibody in a complex antigen system using either the radioimmunoprecipitation (double-antibody) assay (RIP) or the *S. aureus* protein A (Staph A) solid-phase radioimmunoassay (SPRIA). Some potential problems of the RIP are illustrated (upper panel), including (1) differential radioiodination of protein antigens [four closed symbols with 0 to 3 radioactive atoms (internal white circles)] and (2) antigen-limiting conditions leading to nonparallelism and underdetection of certain antibody specificities. The SPRIA (lower panel) avoids radioiodination of antigen mixtures and operates in large antigen excess to avoid the above problems of differential radioiodination and nonparallelism. (Reproduced with permission from Hamilton and Adkinson, 1981.)

criticism of these agents concerns their bulky nature, which tends to reduce immunoreactivity of the labeled ligand or biological activity of labeled cell receptors.

In disciplines where it is necessary to label complex mixtures of proteins (e.g., extracts of allergens or infectious agents), caution should be exercised due to the problems of nonparallelism and differential plateauing that arise from differential labeling (Hamilton and Adkinson, 1981). These problems are depicted schematically in Fig. 2, using a specific antibody immunoassay as an model. Problems associated with the labeling of antigen mixtures can be minimized either by isolating and labeling specific proteins of biological relevance or by using a nonlabeled form of the antigens (solid-phase antigen). Other problems resulting from the radioiodination of proteins involve damage and loss of immunoreactivity of the labeled reagent due to excessive iodination (Izzo *et al.*, 1964), chemical alteration of the ligand following decay of neighboring molecules which can break bonds, the hazard of volatilized iodine at neutral pH levels

(Hamilton and Button, 1980), and radioiodine quality with regard to contaminants (^{124}I, ^{127}I). Loss of immunoreactivity of labeled ligands and receptors following iodination and during storage, however, is a molecule-dependent phenomenon. Labeled protein A from *Staphylococcus aureus,* for example, maintains a high immunoreactivity (>90%) for long periods (up to 10 months), in part due to its stable α-helix structure (Dyrberg and Billestrup, 1984; Wang and Mayer, 1984).

Beta-emitting isotopes (^{14}C and ^{3}H) resolve some concerns about radiation damage of labeled ligands, but they pose other difficulties which involve the use of liquid scintillation cocktail and quench correction algorithms for accurate quantitation. Beta-emitting isotopes continue to be used as labels for a minority of small molecules (e.g., prostaglandin) in both research and clinical ligand binding assays.

B. Nonisotopic Labels

Several attractive features of nonisotopic labels have promoted their wide acceptance among members of the immunoassay community. A long shelf life offers the possibility of standardization and wide distribution of large lots of labeled ligand. The expense of color- and photon-measuring equipment is generally less than that used in radioisotope detection. A detailed review of the nonisotopic alternatives to radiolabels is presented by Schall and Tenoso (1981). Among the most reported nonisotopic labels are enzymes such as horseradish peroxidase (Nakane and Kawsoi, 1974) and alkaline phosphatase, fluorochromes (Gerson, 1984) such as fluorescein isothiocyanate (Colbert *et al.,* 1984), and chemiluminescence labels such as the acridinium esters (Weeks and Woodhead, 1984). Less widely publicized labels include luciferase/ATP conjugates (Carrico *et al.,* 1976) and spin resonance adsorption labels such as the nitroxide radical and 2,4-dinitrophenyl. Two excellent textbooks on the application of enzymes (Maggio, 1980) and luminescent labels (Serio and Pazzagli, 1982) to ligand binding assays provide detailed descriptions of conjugation methods and optimization procedures for multiple assay configurations.

The avidin–biotin system has been used successfully in nonisotopic labeled-antibody immunoassays. It appears to enhance assay sensitivity by increasing the number of labels bound to the detection antibody without disrupting the primary ligand–receptor binding reaction. Biotin is a water-soluble vitamin that is relatively polar and is readily coupled to antibodies under mild conditions that cause little disruption of their structure. Avidin is a tetramer of identical subunits of MW 15,000 that may be coupled to enzymes, fluorochromes, or other labels (Heitzmann and Richards, 1974; Heggeness and Ash, 1977). Because of the high affinity of avidin for biotin (10^{15} liters/mole), avidin-conjugated labels will attach in high number to biotinylated antibody, maximizing the number of tracer molecules bound and the ultimate signal detected. The distinct advantages of these reagents are the low cost of avidin and biotin, the elimination of bulky labeled anti-immunoglobulin molecules, and the use of one avidin-conjugated label for many different immunoassays (Goding, 1983; Liu and Green, 1985).

C. Labeled-Reagent Quality Control

Multiple parameters can be monitored to ensure the quality of labeled ligands and receptors. The specific activity (amount of label per unit mass of ligands or receptor) is one such indicator of quality. Methods used to measure the specific activity of radioiodinated ligands involve column chromatography (Thorell and Larson, 1978), trichloroacetic acid precipitation, immunoassay autodisplacement, and isotope dilution (Englebienne and Sleger, 1983). The column recovery method (protein bound in the void volume versus total activity added to column) and isotope dilution method (displacement of labeled ligand binding to limited binding sites with an equal mass of unlabeled ligand) produce similar specific activity results. The autodisplacement method (comparison of the inhibition produced by the labeled ligand on its own binding to antibody with that produced by unlabeled ligand) gave a higher estimation than the other two methods, presumably because of the presence of immunologically unreactive labeled substances in the labeled-ligand preparation (Englebienne and Sleger, 1983). The specific activity of horseradish peroxidase-conjugated antibodies can be determined in a similar manner by a differential wavelength spectrophotometric method (Sternberger et al., 1970).

V. SEPARATION TECHNIQUES

Immunoassays have been divided into homogeneous assays, which require no physical separation (Rubenstein et al., 1972; Boguslaski and Li, 1982; Looney, 1984), and heterogeneous assays, which require physical separation in order to determine degree of displacement or binding by monitoring the bound/free ratio of labeled ligand or receptor (see Chapter 1). An overview of separation methods most commonly employed in heterogeneous immunoassays is presented in Table IV.

A. Liquid-Phase Methods

Separation of free and bound labeled ligand or receptor was accomplished in many early immunoassays by *differential adsorption* of the labeled reagent to a solid material. Examples of this separation method include the use of cellulose powder (Zaharko and Beck, 1968), dextran-coated charcoal (Odell, 1980), ion-

Table IV. Separation Methods in Heterogeneous Immunoassays

Methods	References
Liquid-phase	
Absorption	
Cellulose powder	Zaharko and Beck, 1968
Dextran-coated charcoal	Odell, 1980
Ion-exchange resin	Lazarus and Young, 1966
Kaolin	Franchimont et al., 1969
QUSO-silica and talc	Rosselin et al., 1966
Nonspecific precipitation	
Alcohol	Makulu et al., 1969
Ammonium sulfate	Chard, 1980
Dioxane	Thomas and Ferin, 1968
Polyethylene glycol	Chard, 1980
Zirconyl phosphate gel	Coffey et al., 1980
Specific precipitation	
Double antibody	Midgley and Hepburn, 1980
Double antibody–PEG	Seibel et al., 1981
Chromatography	
Microfiltration	Chalkley and Renshaw, 1980
Affinity chromatography column	Freytag et al., 1984
Solid-phase	
Mobile	
Agarose beads (Sepharose)	Hamilton et al., 1980
Cellulose disks	Light et al., 1977
Dextran beads (Sephadex)	Wide and Porath, 1966
Ferromagnetic particles	Pourfarzaneh et al., 1982
Gelatin capsule halves	Kerschensteiner, 1984
Latex particles	Masson et al., 1983
Liposomes	Kung and Martin, 1984
Methyl methacrylate particles	Millan et al., 1985
Nylon balls	Djurup, 1983
Polystyrene balls	Ziola et al., 1977
Porous glass beads	Odstrchel, 1980
Erythrocytes	Borsos and Langone, 1983
S. aureus protein A	Lindmark, 1982
Shell/core particles	Litchfield et al., 1984
Stationary	
Capillary tubes	Zick et al., 1980
Cellulose threads	Miller et al., 1984
Chromatography tubes	Pick and Wagner, 1980
Glass rods	Hamaguchi et al., 1976
Indium-coated slide	Giaever, 1973
Microtiter plates	Clark and Engvall, 1980
Nitrocellulose paper	Pappas et al., 1983
Paper–Mylar–polystyrene strips	Walter et al., 1983
Plastic tubes	Catt and Tregear, 1967
Plexiglas [poly(methyl methacrylate)]	Sedlacek et al., 1983

exchange resins (Lazarus and Young, 1966), kaolin (Franchimont *et al.*, 1969), and QUSO-silica and talc (Rosselin *et al.*, 1966) to differentially adsorb unbound labeled ligand. Following sedimentation of the adsorbent, the bound labeled ligand is decanted and free and/or bound fractions are counted for radioisotopic or enzymatic activity or fluorescence. Distinct advantages of this mode of separation are its low cost and ease of separating small ligands from high-molecular-weight receptors. Concerns about misclassification errors resulting from stripping of labeled ligand from receptor and dependence on the time, temperature, buffer, pH, and ionic strength conditions of the assay have caused this modality to become less popular (Jacobs, 1982).

A second liquid-phase method of separation is *nonspecific precipitation,* which involves addition of a salt or a solvent that changes the solubility properties of the receptor–ligand complexes and causes them to precipitate from solution. Reagents used in this method of separation include alcohol (Makulu *et al.*, 1969), ammonium sulfate (Chard, 1980), dioxane (Thomas and Ferin, 1968), polyethylene glycol (PEG) (Chard, 1980), and zirconyl phosphate gel (Coffey *et al.*, 1980). The advantages of low cost, rapidity, and adaptability for automation are offset by the problems of temperature and carrier protein dependence. Caution must be exercised when using these separation methods because of the nonspecific nature of precipitating molecules. Erroneously positive results can be generated in immunoassays that employ polyethylene glycol to precipitate immune complexes, especially in serum containing autoantibodies (e.g., rheumatoid factor) (Hamilton *et al.*, 1984).

Specific precipitation is a third liquid-phase separation method employed in immunoassays. Addition of second antibody (e.g., goat anti-rabbit IgG) causes lattice formation with the primary antibody (rabbit anti-ligand) and immune complexes precipitate. Both preprecipitation (simultaneous addition of both primary and secondary antibodies prior to the addition of labeled and unlabeled ligands) and postprecipitation (addition of second antibody after addition of the ligands) have been successfully employed. The double-antibody mode of separation has the advantage of minimizing misclassification errors by complexing with the primary antibody. The method can be applied to the measurement of a wide spectrum of analyte molecular weights (Midgley and Hepburn, 1980). Second antibody separation tends to be more expensive than the methods discussed above. Incubation times are generally longer than those in other methods, and changing lots of precipitating antibody can make long-term quality control of assays more difficult. Polyethylene glycol may be added to the double-antibody precipitation mixture to increase the rate of reaction and shorten the incubation times required for successful separation of free and bound labeled ligands and receptors (Seibel *et al.*, 1981).

Less widely employed methods of separation include molecular size *chro-*

matography such as microfiltration (Chalkley and Renshaw, 1980), affinity column chromatography (Fretag *et al.*, 1984), and *electrophoresis* (Berson and Yalow, 1973). The major disadvantages of temperature sensitivity, time-consuming manipulations such as packing columns or pouring gels, and difficulty in processing many specimens at one time are cited as reasons for their limited use as separation methods.

B. Solid-Phase Methods

Improved methods for the preparation and synthesis of biopolymers and covalent coupling of receptors and ligands (Scouten, 1983) continue to expand the number of solid phases available for immunoassay separation. Two groups of solid-phase separation methods employed in immunoassays are based on mobile solid-phase reagents (particles free to move in solution) and stationary solid-phase reagents (surfaces on which receptors or ligands have been adsorbed or covalently coupled). When selecting a solid phase for an immunoassay, the assayist should, when possible, select a material that permits the covalent coupling of ligands or receptors onto its surface. This will avoid problems associated with poor absorption onto surfaces due to steric hindrance and electrostatic charge mismatching and will maximize the binding capacity of the sorbent.

1. Mobile Solid-Phase Reagents

Multiple polysaccharide particles such as agarose (Sepharose: Hamilton *et al.*, 1980), cellulose beads (Avicel: Light *et al.*, 1977), paper disks, and dextran beads (Sephadex: Wide and Porath, 1966) have been employed successfully as solid phases for immunoassays. These carbohydrate particles are readily activated with cyanogen bromide to covalently couple protein (Cuatrecasas and Anfinsen, 1971; March *et al.*, 1974). In a comparative study, agarose (a D-galactose-3,6-anhydro-L-galactose polymer) demonstrated a higher binding capacity for antibody than cellulose (D-glucose-1-4-D-glucose) and Sephadex (Yunginger and Gleich, 1972). Naturally occurring human antibodies against cellulose and agarose (Hamilton and Adkinson, 1985) and dextran (Kabat, 1956) have been reported, making it imperative that serum be preabsorbed with the appropriate uncoupled carbohydrate particles prior to assay in immunoassays using one of these solid phases.

One drawback to the use of carbohydrate particles is the requirement for centrifugation. To address this criticism, ferromagnetic particles have been developed which sediment with an electromagnet (Pourfarzaneh *et al.*, 1982). Others investigators have employed adsorption or coupling onto other particle surfaces, including polystyrene beads (Ziola *et al.*, 1977), porous glass beads (Odstrchel, 1980), gelatin capsule halves (Kerschensteiner, 1984), liposomes

(Kung and Martin, 1984), nylon balls (Djurup, 1983), methyl methacrylate particles (Millan *et al.*, 1985), shell/core particles (Litchfield *et al.*, 1984), latex particles (Masson *et al.*, 1983), and red blood cells (Borsos and Langone, 1983). The surface chemistry involved in the derivatization of particles for subsequent covalent coupling can be exemplified by the preparation of surface-derivatized controlled pore glass beads examined by Haller (1983).

Inactivated *S. aureus,* an anaerobic bacterium containing protein A, has become a widely used solid-phase separating reagent for immunoassays (Lindmark, 1982). Protein A is a 42,000-dalton surface protein which binds human IgG subclasses 1, 2, and 4 and many classes of animal immunoglobulins with high affinity (Lind *et al.*, 1970). This specific binding to immunoglobulins permits their extraction from the fluid-phase reaction mixture of an immunoassay and allows the quantitation of free versus antibody-bound labeled ligand (Goding, 1983). The Raji cell provides another example of a cell-bound receptor that has been used to extract complement-fixed immune complexes from serum (Theofilopoulos *et al.*, 1974). Raji cells are human lymphoblast cells that have surface receptors for human complement component 3, which binds some circulating immune complexes.

A novel separation technique employs starch microspheres containing entrapped charcoal and bismuth oxide, which are added to a mixture containing free and bound radiolabeled ligand, e.g., thyroxine (T_4). The charcoal binds unbound radiolabeled ligand and, once centrifuged, the bismuth oxide attenuates the pelleted ^{125}I during γ counting. This assay can achieve a useful working range and acceptable intra- and interassay precision without the need to decant the bound from free activity (Eriksson *et al.*, 1981).

2. Stationary Solid-Phase Reagents

Investigators have employed stationary solid phases in an attempt to eliminate centrifugation, simplify the chemistry of the binding reaction, and automate the assay. Microtechniques of coating antibody on capillary tubes (Zick *et al.*, 1980), glass rods (Hamaguchi *et al.*, 1976), or chromatography tubes (Pick and Wagner, 1980) have not been widely employed. Coating of plastic microtiter plates, tubes, and flat surfaces with antigens or antibodies, however, is widely used (Catt and Tregear, 1967; Clark and Engvall, 1980; Sedlacek *et al.*, 1983). One criticism of coated plastic solid phases concerns the adsorption of molecules onto a surface in a configuration which can mask immunoreactive determinants and reduce immunoreactivity. Plates and tubes also have a limited binding capacity for protein (approximately 1 μg per microtiter well).

A desire to increase the binding capacity, reduce steric hindrance, and minimize immunoreactivity loss when adsorbing onto plastic surfaces has led investigators to experiment with the immobilization of antibody using spacer arms and coupling agents such as toluene 2,4-diisocyanate (Saito, 1983) and glutaraldehyde. None of these techniques thus far has been widely used in clinical or research immunoassays, in part because the most common receptor adsorbed on plastic is antibody, which adsorbs well to plastic surfaces while maintaining most of its immunoreactivity.

More recently, paper (activated and unactivated) has become a solid-phase support for ligand–receptor reactions. Nitrocellulose paper (Pappas *et al.*, 1983) has been configured into a dot-ELISA by fixing antigen covalently and detecting antibody in micro amounts. Whatman 31ET paper fixed with a Mylar–polystyrene backing has been impregnated with drugs for use in fluorescent immunoassays (Walter *et al.*, 1983). Mylar slides coated with a thin layer of indium oxide have been used in an interesting immunoassay configuration which involves a change in visual density with the binding of increasing numbers of antibody and antigen layers (Giaever, 1973). The indium slide immunoassay has permitted a noncompetitive binding reaction of adsorbed antibody with a test ligand under field conditions where immunoassay reactions can be monitored with changes in visual density. Finally, antigens have been covalently coupled to cellulose threads for the purpose of extracting specific antibody from serum. This assay configuration is a novel application of solid-phase technology to potential office, field, or home diagnostics, using film as the detection medium for the signal (counts per minute or fluorescence) (Miller *et al.*, 1984).

VI. BUFFERS

Efficiency of the binding reaction between the receptor and ligand is in part governed by its environment (pH, ionic strength) and the presence of additives (carrier proteins, detergents, proteolytic enzyme inhibitors, and antibacterial chemicals). Table II lists several major buffer systems that have been employed in immunoassays. The buffer salts maintain a restricted pH range and establish the ionic strength. Other additives function in important roles. Tween 20 (1–50 ml per liter of buffer) is added as a detergent to reduce nonspecific binding. Sodium azide (0.01–1 g/liter) prevents bacterial growth during buffer storage and prolonged assay incubations. Bovine and human serum albumin and other proteins (1–10 g/liter) are added to block nonspecific binding sites. In assays where small particles can cause interference (e.g., particle counting assays), the buffer is filtered through a 0.22-μ filter.

Several reports have indicated that the pH of the reaction mixture can significantly affect the performance of peptide hormone immunoassays (Brodsky *et al.*, 1959). This effect on binding of different ionic strengths and pH conditions, however, appears to be unpredictable, as indicated by a systematic study of nonspecific effects in four immunoassays for the measurement of insulin, secretin, gastrin, and human growth hormone (Kajubi *et al.*, 1981). The overall binding and final results of an insulin assay were detectably altered by changes in both the pH and ionic strength, while in a secretin immunoassay run under the same conditions the results remained unaffected. The conclusion of this study was that one cannot *a priori* predict the optimal pH or buffer to be employed in any immunoassay system and that multiple buffer conditions must be examined empirically for each antigen and antiserum combination prior to settling on the "optimal" conditions.

ACKNOWLEDGMENTS

This work was supported in part by grants from the UNDP/World Bank/WHO Special Programme for Research and Training in Tropical Diseases (840489), the National Institutes of Health (AI-19417 and AI-22367), and the Lupus Foundation of America.

REFERENCES

Abraham, G. E., and Grover, P. K. (1971). Covalent linkage of hormonal haptens to protein carriers for use in radioimmunoassay. *In* "Principles of Competitive Protein-Binding Assays" (W. D. Odell and W. H. Daughaday, eds.), pp. 134–140. Lippincott, Philadelphia.

Beisiegel, U., Schneider, W. J., Goldstein, J. L., Andersen, R. G., and Brown M. S. (1981). Monoclonal antibodies to low-density lipoprotein receptor as probes for study of receptor mediated endocytosis and the genetics of familial hypercholesterolemia. *J. Biol. Chem.* **256,** 11923.

Belcher, M. (1984). Receptors, antibodies and disease. *Clin. Chem.* **30,** 1137.

Berne, B. H., Galland, K. T., and Welton, R. C. (1984). Values of the U.S. national reference serum for human antibodies to native DNA obtained with commercial immunoassays for anti-DNA in systemic lupus erythematosus. *Clin. Chem.* **30,** 757.

Berson, S. A., and Yalow, R. S. (1959). Quantitative aspects of reaction between insulin and insulin-binding antibody. *J. Clin. Invest.* **38,** 1996.

Berson, S. A., and Yalow, R. S. (1973). Radioimmunoassay. *In* "Methods in Investigative and Diagnostic Endocrinology. Part I. Methodology" (S. A. Berson and R. S. Yalow, eds.), pp. 84–120. American Elsevier, New York.

Boguslaski, R. C., and Li, T. M. (1982). Homogeneous immunoassays: a review. *Appl. Biochem. Biotechnol.* **7,** 401.

Bolton, A. E., and Hunter, W. M. (1973). The labelling of proteins to high specific radioactivities by conjugation to an I-125 containing acylating agent. *Biochem. J.* **133,** 529.

Borsos, T., and Langone, J. J. (1983). Detection of antigens and haptens by inhibition of passive immune hemolysis. *In* "Methods in Enzymology, Vol. 74, Immunochemical Techniques" (J. J. Langone and H. Van Vunakis, eds.), pp. 161–165. Academic Press, New York.

Brodsky, G. M., Peng, C. T., and Forsham, P. H. (1959). Effect of modification of insulin on specific binding in insulin-resistant sera. *Arch. Biochem. Biophys.* **81,** 1.

Carraway, K. L. (1975). Covalent labelling of membranes. *Biochim. Biophys. Acta* **415,** 379.

Carrico, R. J., Yeung, K., Schroeder, H. R., Boguslaski, R. C., Buckler, R. T., and Christner, J. E. (1976). Specific protein-binding reactions monitored with ligand-ATP conjugates and firefly luciferase. *Anal. Biochem.* **76,** 95.

Catt, K., and Tregear, G. (1967). Solid-phase radioimmunoassay in antibody coated tubes. *Science* **158,** 1570.

Chalkley, S., and Renshaw, A. (1980). Microfiltration as a means of separating free antigen from antigen–antibody complexes in immunoassay. *In* "Methods in Enzymology, Vol. 70, Immunochemical Techniques" (J. J. Langone, ed.), pp. 305–314. Academic Press, New York.

Chard, T. (1980). Ammonium sulfate and polyethylene glycol as reagents to separate antigen from antigen–antibody complexes. *In* "Methods in Enzymology, Vol. 70, Immunochemical Techniques" (J. J. Langone, ed.), pp. 280–290. Academic Press, New York.

Chard, T., ed. (1983). "An Introduction to Radioimmunoassay and Related Techniques." North Holland, New York.

Chase, M. W. (1967). Production of antiserum. *In* "Methods of Immunology and Immunochemistry" (A. Williams and M. W. Chase, eds.), pp. 197–209. Academic Press, New York.

Clark, B. R., and Engvall, E. (1980). Enzyme-linked immunosorbent assay (ELISA): theoretical and practical aspects. *In* "Enzyme-Immunoassay" (E. T. Maggio, ed.), pp. 167–212. CRC Press, Boca Raton, Florida.

Coffey, J., Vandevoorde, J. P., Sauerzopf, E. R., and Hansen, H. J. (1980). Use of zirconyl phosphate gel for the separation of antigen–antibody complexes. *In* "Methods in Enzymology, Vol. 70, Immunochemical Techniques" (J. J. Langone, ed.), pp. 299–305. Academic Press, New York.

Colbert, D. L., Smith, D. S., Landon, J., and Sidki, A. M. (1984). Single-reagent polarization fluoroimmunoassay for barbiturates in urine. *Clin. Chem.* **30,** 1765.

Cuatrecasas, P., and Anfinsen, C. B. (1971). Affinity chromatography. *Methods Enzymol.* **22,** 351.

David, G. S., Wang, R., and Bartholomew, R. (1981). The hybridoma—an immunochemical laser. *Clin. Chem.* **27,** 1580.

Djurup, R. (1983). A nylon ball solid phase radioimmunoassay for specific antibodies in human sera. Application to measurement of IgG antibodies to pollen allergens. *J. Immunol. Methods* **62,** 283.

Duncan, P. H., McKneally, S. S., MacNeil, M. L., Fast, D. M., and Bayse, D. D. (1984). Development of a reference material for alkaline phosphatase. *Clin. Chem.* **30,** 93.

Dyrberg, T., and Billestrup, N. (1984). Preparation of I-125 protein A usable for up to 10 months in immunoassays. *J. Immunol. Methods* **71,** 193.

Eisentraut, A. M., Whissen, N., and Unger, R. H. (1968). Incubation damage in the radioimmunoassay for human plasma glucagon and its prevention with Trasylol. *Am. J. Med. Sci.* **255,** 136.

Ekins, R. P. (1960). The estimation of thyroxine in human plasma by an electrophoretic technique. *Clin. Chim. Acta* **5,** 463–469.

Ekins, R. P. (1974). Basic principles and theory of radioimmunoassay. *Br. Med. Bull.* **30,** 3.

Englebienne, P., and Sleger, G. (1983). Estimation of the specific activity of radioiodinated gonadotropins: comparison of three methods. *J. Immunol. Methods* **56,** 135.

Eriksson, H., Mattiasson, B., and Thorell, J. I. (1981). Use of an internal attenuator in RIA: assay of triiodothyronine (T_3) using starch particles containing entrapped charcoal and bismuth oxide in combination with free antibody. *J. Immunol. Methods* **42,** 105.

Fraker, P. J., and Speck, J. C. (1978). Protein and cell membrane iodinations with sparingly soluble chloroamide 1,3,4,6-tetrachloro-3a-6a-diphenylglycouril. *Biochem. Biophys. Res. Commun.* **80,** 849.

Franchimont, P., Legros, J. J., Deconinck, E., and Brunetti, A. (1969). Separation of free and antibody bound labelled hormone by kaolin in HGH radioimmunoassay. *Horm. Metab. Res.* **1,** 218.

Franchimont, P., Hendrick, J. C., and Reuter, A. M. (1983). Antibody production for immunoassay. *In* "Principles of Competitive Protein Binding Assays" (W. D. Odell and P. Franchimont, eds.), pp. 33–55. John Wiley & Sons, New York.

Fraser, C. M., and Lindstrom, J. (1984). The use of monoclonal antibodies in receptor characterization and purification. *In* "Receptor Biochemistry and Methodology," Vol. 3 (J. C. Venter and L. C. Harrison, eds.), pp. 1–30. Alan R. Liss, New York.

Fraser, C. M., and Venter, J. C. (1982). The size of the mammalian lung B_2 adrenergic receptor as determined by target size analysis and immunoaffinity chromatography. *Biochem. Biophys. Res. Commun.* **109**, 21.

Freytag, J. W., Dickinson, J. C., and Tseng, S. Y. (1984). A highly sensitive affinity-column-mediated immunometric assay, as exemplified by digoxin. *Clin. Chem.* **30**, 417.

Freund, J., and Thomson, H. J. (1948). Antibody formation and sensitization with the aid of adjuvants. *J. Immunol.* **60**, 383.

Gerson, B. (1984). Fluorescence immunoassay. *J. Clin. Immunoassay* 7(1), 73.

Ghanem, G., Legros, F., Lejeune, F., and Fruhling, J. (1982). Comparison and evaluation of different methods for alpha-MSH labelling. *J. Immunol. Methods* **54**, 223.

Giaever, I. (1973). The antibody-antigen reaction: a visual observation. *J. Immunol.* **110**, 1424.

Goding, J. W., ed. (1983). "Monoclonal Antibodies: Principles and Practice. Production and Application of Monoclonal Antibodies in Cell Biology, Biochemistry and Immunology," pp. 56–97. Academic Press, New York.

Greene, G. L., Nolan, C., Engler, J. P., and Jensen, E. V. (1980). Monoclonal antibodies to human estrogen receptor. *Proc. Natl. Acad. Sci. U.S.A.* **77**, 157.

Greenwood, F. C., Hunter, W. M., and Glover, J. S. (1963). The preparation of I-131 labelled human growth hormone of high specific radioactivity. *Biochem. J.* **113**, 299.

Hales, C. N., and Woodhead, J. S. (1980). Labeled antibodies and their use in the immunoradiometric assay. *In* "Methods in Enzymology, Vol. 70, Immunochemical Techniques" (J. J. Langone, ed.), p. 334. Academic Press, New York.

Haller, W. (1983). Application of controlled pore glass in solid phase biochemistry. *In* "Solid Phase Biochemistry: Analytical and Synthetic Aspects" (W. H. Scouten, ed.), pp. 535–597. John Wiley & Sons, New York.

Hamaguchi, Y., Kato, K., Fukui, H., Shirakawa, I., Ishikawa, E., Kobayasi, K., and Katunuma, N. (1976). Enzyme-linked sandwich immunoassay of ornithine delta-aminotransferase from rat liver using antibody coupled glass rods as solid phase. *J. Biochem.* **80**, 895.

Hamilton, R. G. (1980). Radioimmunoassay of human IgG and IgE antibodies. Dissertation, Johns Hopkins Univ. Press, Baltimore.

Hamilton, R. G., and Adkinson, N. F., Jr. (1981). Quantitation of antigen-specific IgG in human serum. II. Comparison of radioimmunoprecipitation and solid phase RIA techniques for the measurement of IgG specific for a complex antigen mixture (yellow jacket venom). *J. Allergy Clin. Immunol.* **67**, 14.

Hamilton, R. G., and Adkinson, N. F., Jr. (1985). Naturally occurring carbohydrate antibodies: interference in solid phase immunoassays. *J. Immunol. Methods* **77**, 95.

Hamilton, R. G., and Adkinson, N. F., Jr. (1987). Quantitative aspects of solid phase immunoassays. *In* "Theoretical and Technical Aspects of ELISA and Other Solid Phase Immunoassays" (M. Kemeny and S. J. Challacombe, eds.). John Wiley & Sons, New York.

Hamilton, R. G., and Button, T. M. (1980). Protein iodination in RIA laboratories: evaluation of commercial ^{125}I-reagents and related biohazards. *J. Immunoassay* **4**, 25.

Hamilton, R. G., and Waud, J. M. (1982). Radioimmunoassay and related methods: Current status and future prospects. *In* "Nuclear Medicine Annual, 1982" (L. M. Freeman and H. S. Weissman, eds.), pp. 225–264. Raven Press, New York.

Hamilton, R. G., Rendell, M., and Adkinson, N. F., Jr. (1980). Serological analysis of human IgG and IgE anti-insulin antibodies using solid phase radioimmunoassays. *J. Lab. Clin. Med.* **96**, 1022.

Hamilton, R. G., Hussain, R., Alexander, E., and Adkinson, N. F., Jr. (1984). Limitations of the radioimmunoprecipitation polyethylene glycol assay (RIPEGA) for detection of filarial antigens in serum. *J. Immunol. Methods* **68**, 349.

Hamilton, R. G., Reimer, C. B., and Rodkey, L. S. (1987). Quality control of murine monoclonal antibodies using isoelectric focusing affinity immunoblot analysis, *Hybridoma* **6**, 205.

Harboe, N., and Ingild, A. (1975). Immunization, isolation of immunoglobulins, estimation of antibody titre. *Scand. J. Immunol.* **2**(1), 161.

Harrison, L. C. (1984). Autoantibodies as probes of receptor structure and function. *In* "Receptor Biochemistry and Methodology, Vol. 2, Receptor Purification Procedures" (J. C. Venter and L. C. Harrison, eds.), pp. 125–139. Alan R. Liss, New York.

Heggeness, M. H., and Ash, J. F. (1977). Use of the avidin–biotin complex for localization of actin and myosin with fluorescence microscopy. *J. Cell Biol.* **73**, 783.

Heitzmann, H., and Richards, F. M. (1974). Use of the avidin–biotin complex for specific staining of biological membranes in electron microscopy. *Proc. Natl. Acad. Sci. U.S.A.* **71**, 3537.

Izzo, J. L., Roncone, A., Izzo, M. J., and Bale, W. F. (1964). Relationship between degree of iodination of insulin and its biological, electrophoretic, and immunochemical properties. *J. Biol. Chem.* **239**, 3749.

Jacobs, P. M. (1982). Separation methods in immunoassay. *J. Clin. Immunoassay* (formerly *Ligand Quarterly*) **5**(1), 1.

Kabat, E. A. (1956). Heterogeneity in the combining regions of human anti-dextran antibody. *J. Immuno.* **77**, 377.

Kabat, E. A., ed. (1976). "Structural Concepts in Immunology and Immunochemistry," 2nd ed. Holt, Rinehart & Winston, New York.

Kajubi, S. K., Yang, R. K., Li, H. R., and Yalow, R. S. (1981). Differential effects of non-specific factors in several radioimmunoassay systems. *J. Clin. Immunoassay* (formerly *Ligand Quarterly*) **4**, 63.

Kerschensteiner, D. (1984). Solid-phase immunoassay using antibody coupled to gelatin capsule halves. *J. Clin. Immunoassay* **7**(1), 61(A).

Kohler, G., and Milstein, C. (1975). Continuous cultures of fused cells secreting antibody of predefined specificity. *Nature (London)* **256**, 495.

Korenman, S. G. (1968). Radio-ligand binding assay of specific estrogens using a soluble uterine macromolecule. *J. Clin. Endocrinol. Metab.* **28**, 127.

Kubasik, N. P., and Sine, H. E. (1976). Serum versus plasma for some substances measured by radioimmunoassay (RIA) techniques. *Clin. Chem.* **22**, 1188.

Kull, F. C., Jr., Jacobs, S., Su, Y. F., and Cuatrecasas, P. (1982). A monoclonal antibody to human insulin receptor. *Biochem. Biophys. Res. Commun.* **106**, 1019.

Kung, V. T., and Martin, F. J. (1984). Liposome-attached ligands enhance agglutination reactions. *J. Clin. Immunoassay* **7**(1), 60A.

Lazarus, L., and Young, J. D. (1966). Radioimmunoassay of human growth hormone using ion exchange resin. *J. Clin. Endocrinol. Metab.* **26**, 213.

Lee, D. S., and Griffiths, B. W. (1984). Comparative studies of iodo-bead and chloramine T methods for the radioiodination of human alpha fetoprotein. *J. Immunol. Methods* **74**, 181.

Light, W., Reisman, R. E., Shimizu, M., and Arbesman, C. E. (1977). Clinical application and measurement of serum levels of bee venom-specific IgE and IgG. *J. Allergy Clin. Immunol.* **59**, 247.

Lind, I., Live, I., and Mansa, B. (1970). Variation in the staphylococcal protein A reactivity with gamma-G globulins of different species. *Acta Pathol. Microbiol. Scand.* **78**, 673.

Lindmark, R. (1982). Fixed protein A-containing staphylococci as solid phase immunoadsorbents. *J. Immunol. Methods,* **52**, 195.

Lindstrom, J., Hochschwender, S., Wan, K., Ratnam, M., and Criado, M. (1985). Use of monoclonal antibodies in exploring the structure of the acetylcholine receptor. *Biochem. Soc. Trans.* **13**, 14.

Litchfield, W. J., Craig, A. R., Frey, W. A., Leflar, C. C., Looney, C. C., and Luddy, M. A. (1984). Novel shell/core particles for automated turbidimetric immunoassays. *Clin. Chem.* **30**, 1489.

Liu, Y. V., and Green, A. (1985). A monoclonal-antibody enzyme immunoassay for detection of hepatitis B surface antigen with use of a biotin–avidin system. *Clin. Chem.* **31,** 202.

Looney, C. E. (1984). High-sensitivity light scattering immunoassays. *J. Clin. Immunoassay* **7**(1), 90.

Maggio, E. T., ed. (1980). "Enzyme Immunoassay." CRC Press, Boca Raton, Florida.

Makulu, Z., Vichick, D., Wright, P. H., Sussman, K. E., and Yu, P. L. (1969). Insulin immunoassay by back-titration using alcohol precipitation of insulin antibody complexes. *Diabetes* **18,** 660.

March, S. C., Parikh, I., and Cuatrecasas, P. (1974). A simplified method for cyanogen bromide activation of agarose for affinity chromatography. *Anal. Biochem.* **60,** 149.

Masson, P. L., Cambiaso, C. L., Collett-Cassart, D., Magnusson, C. M., Richards, C. B., and Sindic, C. M. (1983). Particle counting immunoassay (PACIA). *In* "Methods in Enzymology, Vol 74, Immunochemical Techniques" (J. J. Langone and H. Van Vunakis, eds.), pp. 106–139. Academic Press, New York.

Midgley, A., Jr., and Hepburn, M. R. (1980). Use of the double antibody method to separate antibody bound from free ligand in radioimmunoassay. *In* "Methods in Enzymology, Vol. 70, Immunochemical Techniques" (J. J. Langone, ed.), pp. 266–273. Academic Press, New York.

Millan, J. L., Nustad, K., and Norgaard-Pedersen, B. (1985). Highly sensitive solid phase immunoenzymometric assay for placental and placental-like alkaline phosphatases with a monoclonal antibody and monodisperse polymer particles. *Clin. Chem.* **31,** 54.

Miller, S. P., Marinkovich, V. A., Riege, D. H., Sell, W. J., and Burd, J. F. (1984). Application of the MAST immunodiagnostic system to the determination of allergen specific IgE. *Clin. Chem.* **30,** 1467.

Murphy, B. E. P., Engelberg, W., and Pattee, C. J. (1963). A simple method for the determination of plasma corticoids. *J. Clin. Endocrinol. Metab.* **23,** 293.

Nakane, P. K., and Kawsoi, A. (1974). Peroxidase labeled antibody. A new method of conjugation. *J. Histochem. Cytochem.* **22,** 1084.

Odell, W. D. (1980). Use of charcoal to separate antibody complexes from free ligand in radioimmunoassay. *In* "Methods in Enzymology, Vol. 70, Immunochemical Techniques" (J. J. Langone, ed.), pp. 274–279. Academic Press, New York.

Odell, W. D., and Daughaday, W. H., eds. (1983). "Principles of Competitive Protein Binding Assays." Lippincott, Philadelphia.

Odstrchel, G. (1980). Preparation of controlled pore glass particles for use in immunoassays. *Ann. Acad. Med. Singapore* **9,** 77.

Pappas, M. G., Hajkowski, R., and Hockmeyer, W. T. (1983). Dot enzyme-linked immunosorbent assay (dot-ELISA): a microtechnique for the rapid diagnosis of visceral leishmaniasis. *J. Immunol. Methods* **64,** 205.

Parratt, D., McKenzie, H., Nielsen, K. H., and Cobb, S. J. (1982). Preparation of antisera and radiolabelling. *In* "Radioimmunoassay of Antibody and Its Clinical Applications" (D. Parratt, ed.), pp. 32–53. John Wiley & Sons, New York.

Pick, A., and Wagner, D. (1980). Chromatography tubes: a novel RIA technique. *J. Immunol. Methods* **32,** 275.

Pourfarzaneh, M., Sandy, K., Johnson, C., and Landon, J. (1982). Production and use of magnetizable particles in immunoassay. *J. Clin. Immunoassay* (formerly *Ligand Quarterly*) **5**(1), 41.

Rosselin, G., Assam, R., Yalow, R. S., and Berson, S. A. (1966). Separation of antibody-bound and unbound peptide hormones labeled with I-131 by talcum powder and precipitated silica. *Nature (London)* **212,** 355.

Rubenstein, K. E., Schneider, R. S., and Ullman, E. F. (1972). Homogeneous-enzyme-immunoassay. A new immunochemical technique. *Biochem. Biophys. Res. Commun.* **47,** 846.

Saito, T. (1983). Immobilization of antibody to a plastic surface by toluene 2,4-diisocyanate and its application to radioimmunoassay. *Clin. Chim. Acta* **133,** 301.

Saxena, B. B. (1981). Pregnancy tests: utility of radioreceptor and radioimmunoassay. *J. Clin. Immunoassay* (formerly *Ligand Quarterly*) **4**, 30.

Schall, R. F., and Tenoso, H. J. (1981). Alternatives to radioimmunoassay: labels and methods. *Clin. Chem.* **27**, 1157.

Scouten, W. H. (1983). Solid phase biochemistry: analytical and synthetic aspects. *In* "Chemical Analysis" (P. J. Elving and J. D. Winefordner, eds.), Vol. 66, Chemical Analysis Series. John Wiley & Sons, New York.

Secher, D. S. (1981). Immunoradiometric assay of human leukocyte interferon using monoclonal antibody. *Nature (London)* **290**, 501.

Sedlacek, H. H., Grigat, H., Renk, T., and Seiler, F. R. (1983). The fluorescence immunoassay using plane surface solid phases (FIAPS). *In* "Methods in Enzymology, Vol 74, Immunochemical Techniques" (J. J. Langone and H. Van Vunakis, eds.), pp. 87–105. Academic Press, New York.

Seibel, M., Levesque, L. A., and Traymore, M. L. (1981). A rapid radioimmunoassay for serum leuteinizing hormone using polyethylene glycol and a double antibody method of separation. *Fertil. Steril.* **35**, 36.

Serio, M., and Pazzagli, M., eds. (1982). "Luminescent Assays: Perspectives in Endocrinology and Clinical Chemistry," Serono Symposia, Vol. 1. Raven Press, New York.

Shively, J. E. (1984). Monoclonal antibodies to CEA. *J. Clin. Immunoassay* **7**, 112.

Sternberger, L. A., Hardy, P. H., Cuculis, J. J., and Meyer, H. G. (1970). The unlabeled antibody enzyme method of immunochemistry. Preparation and properties of soluble antigen–antibody complex (horseradish peroxidase–anti-horseradish peroxidase) and its use in the identification of spirochetes. *J. Histochem. Cytochem.* **18**, 315.

Theofilopoulos, A. N., Dixon, F. J., and Bokisch, V. A. (1974). Binding of soluble immune complexes to human lymphoblastoid cells. I. Characterization of receptor for IgG Fc and complement and description of the binding mechanism. *J. Exp. Med.* **140**, 877.

Thomas, K., and Ferin, J. (1968). A new rapid radioimmunoassay for HCG (LH, ICSH) in plasma using dioxan. *J. Clin. Endocrinol. Metab.* **28**, 1667.

Thorell, J. I., and Johansson, B. G. (1971). Enzymatic iodination of polypeptides with I-125 to high specific activity. *Biochim. Biophys. Acta* **251**, 363.

Thorell, J. I., and Larson, S. M., eds. (1978). "Radioimmunoassay and Related Techniques: Methodology and Clinical Applications." C. V. Mosby, St. Louis.

Trowbridge, I. S., and Lopez, F. (1982). Monoclonal antibody to transferrin receptor blocks transferrin binding and inhibits human tumor cell growth *in vitro*. *Proc. Natl. Acad. Sci. U.S.A.* **79**, 1175.

Updyke, T. V., and Nicolson, G. L. (1984). Immunoaffinity isolation of membrane antigens with biotinylated monoclonal antibodies and immobilized streptavidin matrices. *J. Immunol. Methods* **73**, 83.

Walter, B., Greenquist, A. C., and Howard, W. E., III (1983). Solid-phase reagent strips for detection of therapeutic drugs in serum by substrate-labeled fluorescent immunoassay. *Anal. Chem.* **55**, 873.

Wang, H. P., and Mayer, P. C. (1984). Immonochemical evaluation of radioiodinated protein A. *J. Immunol. Methods* **72**, 61.

Weeks, I., and Woodhead, J. S. (1984). Chemiluminescence immunoassay. *J. Clin. Immunoassay* **7**(1), 82.

Wide, L., and Porath, J. (1966). Radioimmunoassay of proteins with the use of Sephadex-coupled antibodies. *Biochim. Biophys. Acta* **130**, 257.

Yavin, E., Yavin, Z., Schneider, M. D., and Kohn, L. D. (1981). Monoclonal antibodies to the thyrotropin receptor: implications for receptor structure and the action of autoantibodies in Graves disease. *Proc. Natl. Acad. Sci. U.S.A.* **78**, 3180.

Yunginger, J. W., and Gleich, G. J. (1972). Comparison of the protein binding capacities of cyanogen bromide-activated polysaccharides. *J. Allergy* **50**, 109.

Zaharko, D. S., and Beck, L. (1968). Studies of a simplified plasma insulin immunoassay using cellulose powder. *Diabetes* **17,** 444.

Zick, R., Schweer, H. H., Mitzkat, H. J., and Frieder, R. (1980). Capillary radioimmunoassay for insulin. *Eur. J. Nucl. Med.* **5,** 423.

Ziola, B. R., Matikainen, M. T., and Salmi, A. (1977). Polystyrene balls as the solid phase of a double antibody radioimmunoassay for human serum albumin. *J. Immunol. Methods* **17,** 309.

Chapter 3

Practical Guide to Immunoassay Method Evaluation

Carolyn S. Feldkamp

Ligand Assay Laboratory
Henry Ford Hospital
Detroit, Michigan 48202

Stuart W. Smith

Nuclear Medicine Service
Veterans Administration Hospital
Allen Park, Michigan 48101

I. INTRODUCTION

Selection of an analytical method which meets the clinical laboratory's objectives of reliable, accurate, timely, and cost-effective service is essential. Evaluation of immunoassays requires an efficient protocol and objective criteria for method selection. A data base is also established for long-term quality control monitoring and troubleshooting. Even when a laboratory uses kits, an understanding of the basic biochemistry involved and how individual components interact contributes to the selection process. Although certain assumptions and constraints are inherent in the use of kits, the experiments that follow are designed to obtain maximum information about performance and the underlying biochemistry.

An overall scheme for systematically testing various aspects of method performance will be described. The protocol can easily be modified, depending on the specific questions being asked, the resources available for the evaluation, and the limitations imposed by the format of the method itself.

Various specific experimental approaches test the performance of a method and whether it meets the defined goals. Appropriate application of the tests described here depends on a thorough understanding of the analytic and biochemical principles involved in the use of the antigen–antibody reaction. Each reagent, separation technique, and method of detecting the label contributes to the final measurement of the unknown analyte. Examination of various data reduction methods is an important tool in the evaluation procedure and a source of misunderstanding as well. The reader is referred to Chapter 1 for background discussion.

A. Specific Laboratory Objectives for Method Evaluation

Before evaluating a new method or starting a new test, preliminary considerations must address the questions, ''Do I want to do the test at all?'' and ''Which methods will I consider?''

To establish the clinical need, potential new information is compared with that available from existing tests, the anticipated ordering pattern, and the number of requests expected. Does the new test have the potential for applications other than the original use? The test should be performed frequently enough to provide the service required in terms of timing and turnaround, while remaining cost-effective. Are there alternative technologies?

The laboratory now has the formidable task of selecting the methods to be evaluated. New methods with convenient timing may result in efficient turn-around and affect overall service by reducing the number of other laboratory tests ordered or repeated. Some methods offer increased sensitivity and specificity, highly purified or unique standards, or easy-to-use formats.

B. Analytical Objectives

The analytical terms ''precision,'' ''accuracy,'' ''sensitivity,'' and ''specificity'' have well-defined meanings in analytical and clinical chemistry, but because of the unique characteristics of immunoassays, these concepts can be complex. Although these concepts are separated here for discussion, they are interrelated. For example, both accuracy and assay sensitivity may be limited by precision. In the current context analytical sensitivity and specificity are distinguished from the concepts of clinical sensitivity and specificity, which are related to the ability to detect the presence or absence of disease (Galen and Gambino, 1975). All of the components of a method—antibody, tracer, analyte, and matrix—interact to contribute to a varying degree to the different performance characteristics.

Assay characteristics described above are analytical goals shared by all clinical laboratories. How well an assay achieves them depends on the unique characteristics of the reagents and on experimental optimization. This chapter will detail specific experiments which allow the immunoassay kit user to assess these qualities in his or her own laboratory.

II. PROTOCOL OUTLINE

A. Objectives and preparation for evaluation
B. Precision
C. Standard curves: shape, data reduction, matrix, interferences
D. Tracer: B_0, immunoreactivity, specific activity
E. Sensitivity
F. Accuracy: parallelism, recovery, cross-reactivity
G. Scatchard plot
H. Clinical validation

III. ESTABLISHING OBJECTIVES AND PREPARATION

A. Protocol Review

The first step is to read the manufacturer's claim carefully. This statement is equivalent to one's mother's reminder to wear galoshes, but a great deal of trouble can be avoided and questions answered before a single reagent is pipetted.

A thorough review of the protocol includes careful attention to timing, temperature, and centrifuge (there is a difference between 3000 rpm and 3000 rcf!). Do reagents need to be prepared fresh? Is decanting or aspiration of supernatants specified? Are the reagents supplied in convenient and economical volumes? Does the format allow the use of repeating pipettes? The following information is generally provided by the manufacturer in the package insert.

1. Precision

Compare claims of precision between kits. Surprisingly, you may have to check the calculations.

2. Standard Curves

Standard curves are usually illustrated. Sensitivity, range, and shapes can be compared by plotting data from different kits on the same scale. This simple procedure may uncover strengths or weaknesses of one kit or another, which may then be investigated further (Garrett, 1985). Considerations include: Are the stated ranges reasonable for the expected clinical samples? Is there a clear distinction between normal range and abnormal patients? Where on the curve do the clinically relevant ranges fall? For example, when the normal range is very near one end of the standard curve, there can be little discrimination within the range.

Normal range statistics may be limited by the sensitivity of the test and normal/abnormal cutoffs may depend on a single standard point in a relatively imprecise part of the curve. Radioimmunoassays (RIAs) of tumor markers such as carcinoembryonic antigen (CEA) or prostatic acid phosphatase often fall in the category of assays in which, though the concentrations observed in patients fall in a very wide range, precise discrimination or quantitation of high values is not always required. On the other hand, precision and sensitivity of the curve in the region of the upper limit of normal are extremely important.

3. Reagents

Information on the source and chemical structure of the antigens, antibodies, and tracers can be related to the specificity expected and can direct attention to certain problems which may be anticipated. The questions a user asks about the reagents vary with the analyte and the anticipated clinical use of the result.

a. Antibody. What animal was used for the first and second antibodies? Is carrier nonimmune serum added to the reaction system?

b. Antigen. What was the antigen? If a hapten conjugate was used, what conjugation method and what carrier protein were used? The length of spacer molecule and point of attachment may be important to the specificity of steroid RIA. Are cross-reacting molecules likely to be present in the sample assayed?

c. Tracer. Is the tracer identical to the standard? Does the conjugate have the same connecting structure as that used in the antigen? Is the tracer purified after labeling? New methods of high-performance liquid chromatography (HPLC) or affinity column chromatography have substantially improved the purity and thus the specific activity and shelf life of some tracers currently on the market.

d. Standard. Is the standard homogeneous, pure, and chemically identical to the unknown to be measured? Can the mass of standard be related to an international standard or reference preparation? What matrix is used? Is enough zero standard included in the kit for dilutions?

B. Information and Planning

Consultation with other users of a method and review of its performance in proficiency surveys and quality control programs provide moral support and a consensus of its popularity, precision, and any systematic bias. It must be kept in mind, however, that consensus alone does not prove accuracy or reliability. The laboratory's own experience with a manufacturer with regard to service, reagent quality, stability, etc. is also frequently an important factor in the final choice.

To evaluate a kit efficiently and to make objective comparisons between methods, adequate quality control materials, standards, and previously assayed samples should be obtained and stored in aliquots. It is impossible to collect sufficient data for comparison if the lot of quality control material changes in the middle of the evaluation. Since highly purified materials or international standards used to test accuracy are often difficult to prepare accurately, or are unstable and expensive, it is often preferable to do recovery comparisons on all methods at the same time, using identical, fresh samples. Patient samples in specified ranges as well as normal controls must be accumulated. Again, plan for the entire evaluation.

Test more than one lot of reagents. To see optimal performance, use fresh radioactive tracer. This condition should show the best sensitivity and maximum precision. Save some tracer until near the expiration date to repeat selected tests with old tracer. Although seldom revealed in the short time of an evaluation, tracer impurity and instability are among the most frequent sources of poor quality control and assay unreliability.

IV. EVALUATION OF PRECISION

Precision is a statistical index of the ability of an assay to yield the same result when the assay is repeated on the same sample. Alternatively, we express this property in terms of the "confidence" we have in a single result. In some clinical contexts the reproducibility of an answer is more important to the physician following the clinical course of a patient than the absolute accuracy of the answer (Garrett and Krouwer, 1985).

A. Definitions

1. Within-run precision. Within-run precision is defined as the precision of the same sample run several times in the same assay. This is a baseline for long-term quality control. Poor within-run precision and front-to-back drift can be due to methodological variations such as poor control of timing steps or not adhering to recommendations for heating or cooling.

2. Between-run precision. Between-run precision is an index of the ability of the assay to reproduce a result on the same sample from day to day, or the confidence interval about a single result.

Both of these measurements are typically done early in the evaluation protocol since, if a method cannot give reproducible results in a given laboratory, it is unlikely that other aspects of the evaluation will be valid or that the method will be acceptable for routine use. A well-planned evaluation with pooled samples prepared to run many times can efficiently accumulate adequate data within and between runs to assess the precision of the kit.

B. Protocol for Precision Studies

1. Materials

Lyophilized quality control pools have the advantages that they are readily available in sufficient quantities and at different concentrations. Data accumulated can form the initial bases for a quality control program. Vial-to-vial variation in lyophilized materials can be avoided by reconstituting enough for the entire evaluation and then freezing one-assay-sized aliquots. It is important, however, that precision also be tested on real samples. Although lyophilized materials are very useful for long-term monitoring, their behavior in immunoassays is not always identical with that of patients' sera. Fresh samples are often more stable and results are more precise than those obtainable on reconstituted serum.

2. Concentrations to Use

Samples for precision studies are usually used in at least three concentrations. Generally the levels selected represent low (80% B_0), midrange (50% B_0 or ED_{50}),[1] and high (20% B_0) doses on the standard curve. If the curve is centered about the normal range, these also represent abnormally low, normal, and abnormally high concentrations in patients. For some tests additional concentrations may be selected to establish the precision in concentration ranges that are of particular clinical interest, such as an abnormal/normal cutoff, or to evaluate a portion of the standard curve for which commercial controls are not available.

3. Calculations

Each of the selected test samples is assayed in two or more replicates in every run. Results are obtained from the standard curve and tabulated. Calculate the mean ($\bar{x}$) and standard deviation (s) for each sample according to the following:

$$\bar{x} = \frac{\Sigma x}{N}$$

and

$$s = \sqrt{\Sigma(x-\bar{x})^2/(N-1)}$$

The calculated standard deviation will be a better estimate of its true value if at least 20 observations are included between and within runs. Practically speaking, $n = 10$ is often used to estimate the within-run precision initially. Since running many replicates in an assay is quite costly in time and materials, an estimate of standard deviation can be made by pooling results on duplicates of individual samples according to the formula (Henry et al., 1974)

[1] B_0 is the binding of the zero standard, the maximum binding. ED_{50} is the estimated dose at 50% of B_0, usually the most sensitive part of the curve.

$$s = \sqrt{(\Sigma d^2)/N}$$

where d is the difference between duplicates and N the number of observations. Since variance in immunoassays is dose-dependent, only data within the same dose range should be pooled for this estimate.

4. Acceptable Performance

A question often asked is, "What is acceptable precision?" High precision is particularly important in the concentration range of critical clinical decisions. Certainly a single laboratory should get standard deviations as low as, or less than, those stated by the reagent manufacturer. Expected ranges stated in quality control product specifications are based on data pooled from several laboratories and are thus much broader than ranges that can be achieved in a single laboratory. Published ranges are helpful only to establish the presence or absence of significant bias compared to others using the same kit. In our experience <10% coefficient of variation (CV) is achievable with most RIA kits.

C. Precision Profile

The response (bound label or some function of bound label) measured in immunoassays is nonlinear and the variance is nonuniform; that is, the precision is different at different analyte concentrations. This is called heteroscadasticity. Imprecision associated with the standard curve reflects the sum of random errors contributed by individual idiosyncrasies and environmental and reagent-related variation. In addition, imprecision is inherent in the underlying biochemical reaction—the saturable, equilibrium reaction. Systematic bias such as that caused by improper standardization or nonspecific antisera is not detected by precision studies.

A device for expressing overall performance is the "precision profile," a graph of coefficient of variation against concentration of analyte (Ekins, 1981). In its simplest form the precision profile is created by assaying many replicates of standards and plotting the CV against the known concentrations. The performance over the entire curve and any existing heteroscadasticity can be visualized (Fig. 1). The shape of this curve changes with any of the methodological or environmental changes which are known to affect precision. These curves may also be used to establish the working range of a kit by clearly indicating the concentrations beyond which the assay precision is unacceptable. Comparisons of different kits, data reduction methods, and the effect of age on kit tracers are all amenable to the use of precision profiles.

Experts differ on when it is preferable to expend resources to prepare the precision profile, since an accurate determination of CV at many doses requires many observations. A complete study is most appropriately done by the manu-

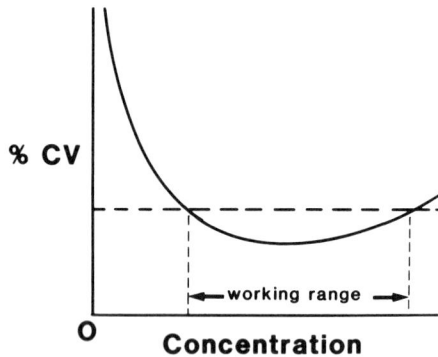

Figure 1. Precision profile. The coefficient of variation is plotted against concentration. When minimal acceptable precision can be defined (dotted line), the working range is defined. (Adapted from Ekins, 1981.)

facturer, where reagents are easily available, and at a time when the assay reagents and conditions are being optimized.

A more practical alternative for constructing a precision profile is to use the observed precision of duplicates of many samples (expressed in terms of CV of calculated dose) plotted against the mean calculated dose (Ekins, 1981). Clearly, this approach is not ideal since the dose axis is not independent; it is based on measurement in the assay being tested. To calculate the CV for the CV versus dose graph, observations on patients are grouped or "binned" into dose ranges and the mean concentration and mean CV used for the profile. Graphs such as these are of the type used in sophisticated computers which weight standard curve points by "historical" precision observations for the purpose of curve fitting.

D. Sources of Imprecision

Aside from assessing precision, it is important during evaluation to reduce both random and systematic errors to the minimum by adherence to the manufacturer's procedures and by careful calibration and quality control of all instruments in the laboratory. A thorough understanding of how individual components, assay conditions, separation techniques, and data reduction methods affect the observed precision of the assay will contribute to a rational review of the method performance and, hopefully, to the ultimate satisfaction of the user (Tables I and II).

1. Kit Components and Protocol

Although the selection of antibody, separation method, and method design and optimization are out of the control of the user, the effect of these choices is felt by the laboratory.

Table I. Source of Variation (Random and/or Systematic)

Source of error	Effect on assay
Pipetting	Accuracy
	Precision
	Carryover
Separation	Reagents
	Reaction
	Timing
	Stripping
	NSB effects
Chemistry	Reagents
	Reaction (equilibrium vs. nonequilibrium)
Counting	Total counts
	Instrumental QC
	Geometry
	Quench
Color reaction	Interference
	Stability

a. Antibody/Binder. Precision is affected by the equilibrium constant (K_{eq}), the rate of reaction (including the effect of antibody concentration, temperature, etc.), and whether equilibrium has been reached (i.e., sequential addition of tracer).

b. Separation Technique. The free and bound fractions should be separated completely and without disruption of the specific binding; that is, there are minimal "misclassification errors." The ideal separation is 100% and instantaneous. Polyethylene glycol (PEG) precipitates or charcoal pellets may be unstable. Incomplete decantation, drops of supernatant left on the side of the test tube, and reaction mixtures which are too concentrated or are in too small a

Table II. Sources of Error: Nonisotopic Assays

Source of error	Effect on assay
Interferences	Add color or reduce color: bilirubin, drugs
	Act as enzyme: hemoglobin, endogenous alkaline phosphatase
	Inhibit enzyme: metals
	Scatter light: lipids, macromolecules
Color reaction	Stability of substrate
	Colored product
Precision	Timing
	Washing
	Separation
	Spectrophotometric error
	Binding reaction

volume to be decanted all reflect poor kit design. Also, some nonspecific interferences such as lipemia affect the separation.

c. Isolation/Extraction Steps. Steps in the procedure such as boiling, acid extraction, or organic solvent extraction add further opportunity for random and systematic errors. Each such procedure should be checked for accuracy or completeness of recovery.

2. Environmental Effects

Immunoassays are more sensitive to small differences in time and temperature than is often realized, resulting in increased CV of quality controls and patient replicates or in unaccountable shifts in controls. Users usually assume that the assays are robust to normal variations in the environment such as the difference in "room temperature" between summer and winter. Since reaction times in kits are often shortened to offer improved turnaround time, true equilibrium cannot be assumed and reaction times must be kept within specified limits. The timing of reagent additions, centrifugation time and speed, and cooling steps may also be critical to maintain precision.

3. Detection of Label

Since radioactive decay is a statistically well-characterized physical event, the errors associated with detecting these tracers are easily assessable and can be reduced to any practical level simply by accumulating sufficient counts in each sample. The standard deviation of counting a single sample (counting error) is equal to the square root of counts accumulated. The common recommendation to count 10,000 counts reduces the counting error to 1%, which can be considered negligible relative to other experimental errors. However, high samples in an assay may bind only a few hundred counts per minute and counting error may contribute significantly to the total assay error. The geometry of the sample in the detector, counter calibration, and background counts also affect random error. Nonisotopic tracers contribute to total error by factors related to the spectrophotometric measurement itself. For these assays, timing of the incubations and reagent addition, stability of the final color, and instrument quality and quality control must also be taken into account.

V. STANDARD CURVES

A. Data Reduction Models

An introduction to the chemical and mathematical principles underlying the competitive binding reaction and the generation of standard curves has been presented in Chapter 1. Different curves tend to highlight different parts of the curve range and in some instances point up situations where the actual chemical behavior of the reaction deviates from the ideal model. It is instructive to plot standard curve data in several ways. A plot of B/T (cpm in the bound fraction divided by total cpm added) versus log dose is sigmoidal and may show a dose range which has poor dose–response (flat) and is thus unusable. The hyperbolic B/F versus dose curve is steep at low concentrations and may be used to compare low-end sensitivity among kits. The logit–log plot linearizes many, but not all, immunoassay curves. Before a data reduction method is selected for day-to-day use, the curve should be evaluated as carefully as other aspects of kit performance to ascertain that the mathematics used fits the standard points well. Poor curve fit can be a substantial source of inaccuracy and imprecision.

B. Standards

The manufacturer's brochure will describe the chemical nature of the standard used, whether it is identical to the analyte, is an analog, a metabolite, or a cross-reacting ligand. For example, RIAs for gastrin employ a synthetic G-17 as a standard and tracer to measure predominantely the larger G-37 and other forms of the hormone. For other analytes (e.g., digoxin), hapten conjugates are used as antigen and as tracer, but the unconjugated molecule is the standard. Standards of complex proteins may be derived from a single tissue, e.g., spleen ferritin or tumor cell CEA, but the assays are expected to measure similar, but not identical, molecules derived from other tissues.

Standards of some hormone assays are related to specific international standards and others are calibrated in mass units. Since secondary standards (kit standards) are not necessarily calibrated against the same reference material and the responses of the standards measured by a unique antibody are not necessarily parallel either to different reference materials or to each other, some methods are difficult to compare.

The selection of particular standard concentrations also affects the usefulness of a particular curve. Are the normal or abnormal ranges of interest located in the most precise and sensitive part of the curve? Is the highest kit standard useful? Large gaps between two adjacent standards should be closely scrutinized. Although for economy one would not want to run an excess of standards, during the evaluation one should dilute the standards provided and fill gaps to ascertain the true shape of the curve. Occasionally this practice will reveal an inflection point between two standards which is not adequately predicted by the curve-fitting algorithm. Point-to-point or spline curve-fitting methods which do not weight points and are not dependent on a chemical model might result in significant inaccuracy in patient results (Fig. 2). The placement of standards near concentrations of particular clinical interest increases the reliability of dose estimates of unknown samples. When unweighted curve-fitting algorithms are used, inclusion of standards which exceed the capacity of the antibody, either high or low,

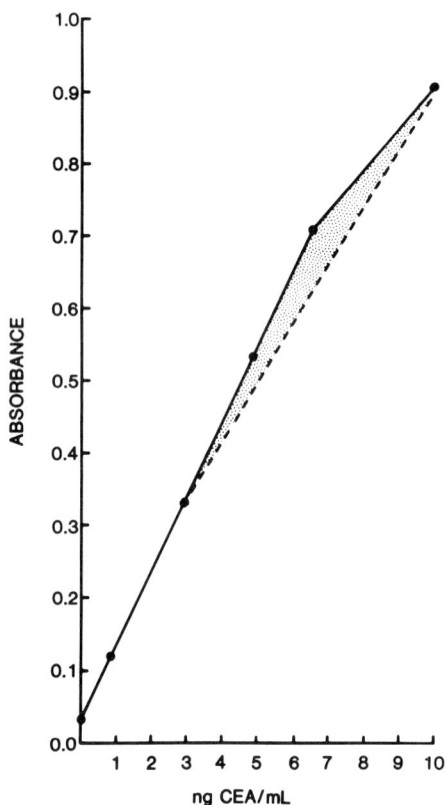

Figure 2. Effect of standard points on accurate dose estimate. For an enzyme immunoassay, a point-to-point curve using 0, 1, 3, and 10 ng/ml standards (dotted line) is recommended. Additional standards, 5 and 6.5 ng/ml, showed a different inflection (Homsher, 1985).

contributes to poor fit of the remainder of the points. If extreme points are truly not useful, then a laboratory may elect to drop them in favor of a standard which is more helpful.

The concentration of the lowest standard is of particular interest. Run one or two dilutions of the lowest standard to verify the linearity and precision near zero. This step is essential if any results below the lowest standard are to be reported. This low-end curve can also be used to evaluate tracer mass and the least detectable dose, as described later.

Occasionally, patient samples or dilutions of standards to very low concentrations produce bound counts which are greater than those in the zero standard (B_0, maximum binding tube). There may be several explanations for this: imprecision of the B_0, or the fact that the zero standard does not adequately reflect the nonspecific binding in a real sample. The curve may also exhibit a shape which is

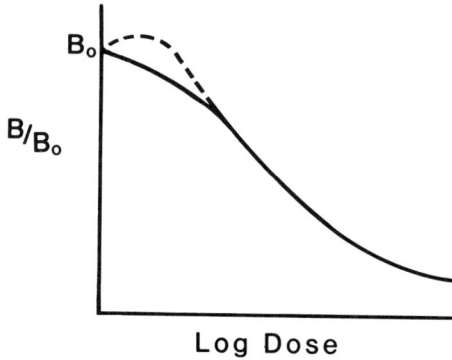

Figure 3. Low-dose hook. Standard curve binding greater than B_0 (dotted line) between the lowest standard and the zero standard.

called a "low-dose hook" (Fig. 3). The characteristic shape has been attributed to positive cooperativity between antigen binding sites on the same antibody or to the formation of stable antibody–ligand rings (Ehrlich and Moyle, 1984). Low-dose hooks can be observed in RIA kits, especially hapten assays in which the tracer can be labeled to a very high specific activity.

A similar-appearing "high-dose hook" seen in IRMA assays and certain nephelometric immunoassays is due to a completely different mechanism (Fig. 4). The hook is analogous to the condition of antigen excess of classical immunoprecipitain assays. Very high levels of antigen saturate antibody binding sites (often solid-phase) and subsequently inhibit proportional binding of a labeled second antibody by binding to the label in solution. When evaluating IRMA methods, patient samples in the highest concentrations to be expected in clinical situations should be assayed at several dilutions to test for the possibility of this hook and avoid the possibility of inaccurately low results (Hoffman, 1985).

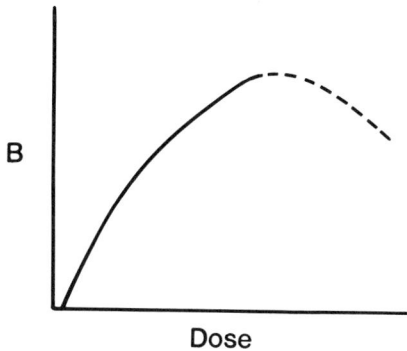

Figure 4. High-dose hook. Decreased binding at high concentrations in IRMA (dotted line).

C. Control Tubes

There is more to a standard curve than standards. Control tubes such as the maximum binding (B_0), nonspecific binding, and other blanks must be included for use in calculations and for correction of nonspecific effects, or "misclassification" errors. The accuracy of the results obtained and the fit of the curves depend on the correct choice of blank or other control tubes, that is, the extent to which any assumptions made about nonspecific matrix effects correspond to reality.

1. Total Counts

A total counts tube contains the total tracer added to each subsequent reaction tube. In calculating the free fraction (total − bound), the assumption is implicit that all of the label is immunoreactive, that is, that the tracer has not been damaged and could bind in the presence of an excess of antibody (see Sec. VI,A,2).

2. Maximum Binding

The maximum binding tube (B_0, zero standard) contains the complete complement of antibody, tracer, "sample" (identical to the sample but without the analyte of interest), and separation medium. B_0 depends on the relative titer of antiserum and tracer, usually adjusted so that B_0 is 30–50% of the total counts. This typical proportion should yield an adequate slope for good sensitivity and a high enough count rate for good precision. Some data reduction methods normalize bound counts in each reaction tube by dividing by B_0. Even when this is recommended, the total counts tube and the B_0 as a percentage of the total counts should be monitored as evidence of tracer stability and immunoreactivity. When B/B_0 or logit B/B_0 is used, the entire standard curve relies on the accuracy and appropriateness of the zero as a control tube. Occasionally the zero is not the same serum as the matrix used in the rest of the standards, but is specially selected and tested to be sure that the binding is always greater than that of true negative patients.

3. Nonspecific Binding

The nonspecific binding (NSB) tube is included in standard curves to account for all tracer which appears in the bound fraction but which does not represent specific, antibody binding. Theoretically, this blank tube should contain everything, including the sample, except the antibody. Nonimmune animal serum replaces the specific antibody. If a kit format allows it, the NSB tube usually contains the tracer, a protein-containing buffer to replace the antiserum, and the sample. The NSB, as a percentage of total counts, should be minimal, that is, a few percent. An alternative correction occasionally recommended is the binding of tracer to antibody observed with cold ligand in excess. This controls for NSB when antibody is in the tube. The tube includes tracer, antibody, $100\times$ the highest standard, and the separation medium. This is rarely done since it is often costly (or impossible) to obtain large amounts of unlabeled standard.

These typical controls correct for tracer bound to the test tube or trapped in pellets but do not account for the nonspecific binding to molecules (especially proteins) introduced from the patient's serum, nor can they correct for loss of immunoreactivity (plasma damage) caused by exposing the tracer to serum enzymes during the binding reaction. The latter effect is more common with low-affinity antibodies, which demand relatively high sample concentrations and long incubation times to achieve sensitivity. However, it is desirable to run patient blanks during the evaluation to verify that the NSB tube does appropriately estimate the true nonspecific binding present in the patient samples. A patient blank contains sample, tracer, buffer or nonimmune serum to replace antibody, and the separation medium. In assays in which a patient blank is shown to be important, each dilution should be corrected with a blank using the same serum dilution. Current methods rarely require patient blanks, but on occasion a variable blank will be observed. This behavior alone may be reason to reject one method in favor of another. Finally, even if no increased blank is observed initially, the possibility of underlying nonspecific binding in the patient sample which is not accounted for by the usual standard blanks should be kept in mind, especially when dilutions of patient samples do not agree. Unusual and unpredictable binding in the presence of patient serum proteins occasionally occurs.

D. Matrix

The matrix of the standard curve is defined as everything in the standard (or sample) that is not the analyte. The main components affecting the antigen–antibody reaction appear to be proteins—their concentration and, in some cases, the specific distribution of individual proteins. For example, it has been found that albumin alone is not an adequate substitute for serum as a matrix for standards in many radioimmunassays. Also of influence in the matrix are pH, ionic strength, and other serum components such as lipids and specific ions. In patients, abnormal levels of specific proteins, immunoglobulins, or enzymes change the matrix. Matrix components affect the separation step as well as the binding reaction. For example, PEG separations are often found to be relatively sensitive to patient-to-patient variation in protein composition.

The standard matrix selected is a material in which the standard reacts with the antibody in the same way as an unknown sample. The matrix should be identical in all standards including the zero standard. The matrix does not have to be human serum, but each antibody must be tested to demonstrate that no shift in the standard curve occurs between standards in human serum and standards in the matrix chosen. Thyrotropin (TSH) is an example of an assay that frequently shows significant differences depending on the matrix used. TSH-free human serum is difficult to obtain and even then it may vary from lot to lot. Although certain animal sera have been used successfully with some antisera (Golstein and Vanhaelst, 1973), the trend toward incorporation of human serum in standard curves has contributed to an overall increase in sensitivity of these assays and consequent lowering of the normal range (Durham, 1985).

1. Patient Sample Interferences

Most manufacturers specify any known interfering substances as well as the acceptable sample preparation. There is usually a general caveat to avoid lipemia and hemolysis.

Specific and nonspecific interferences often influence the blank correction such that the usual NSB does not adequately correct for all the "bound fraction" not attributable to the specific antibody. Some substances inhibit tracer binding directly and others may increase the underlying blank by specifically or non-specifically binding the tracer. In nonisotopic assays interfering substances may add directly to the detected signal, e.g., color, enzymatic activity, reducing power, or turbidity.

Some substances such as lipids influence the separation step, reducing the precision and accuracy of the assay by interfering with the formation of precipitates with a second antibody or PEG. Note should be made when a particular type of nonspecific interference is common in the population to be tested with a particular assay. For example, an assay for prostatic acid phosphatase which is very sensitive to the presence of lipids, might be expected to have a high frequency of problems since the test would be used to evaluated middle-aged and older men, a population which also shows an increased frequency of elevated serum lipids.

Proteins are frequently reported to be specific and nonspecific interferences. Natural binding proteins can bind tracer and increase or decrease the final result depending on the separation method. Familial alterations in albumin binding are reported to interfere in some free T_4 assays (Stockigt et al., 1983). An often overlooked problem is the presence in the patient sample of antibodies directed toward some component of the reaction mixture. Among these endogenous anti-insulin developed in diabetics taking bovine or porcine insulin was an important problem in the radioimmunoassay for insulin (Feldkamp et al., 1977). The magnitude of the effect depended on the separation method used. With dextran-coated charcoal the bound fraction was increased by tracer bound to patient antibodies and the results were too low and not parallel on dilution. With second antibody separations, the result could be erroneously high, depending on the blank correction. Recently, occasional problems have been reported which have been traced to the presence of anti-rabbit antibodies in patient sera (Gendrel *et al.*, 1981; Vladutiu *et al.*, 1982). In some TSH assays, if there is not enough carrier rabbit serum, the patient's antibodies to animal proteins inhibit the binding of antigen to the specific antibody, resulting in spuriously high results.

2. Diluents

The selection of a suitable diluent for high samples requires many of the same considerations as in the previous discussion of matrix and blanking and a variety of buffered protein solutions have been used (Table III). We attempt to assay the unknown sample in the most precise and accurate part of the standard curve and expect the result to be independent of the amount of serum assayed, that is, dilutions to be parallel to the standard curve. The best diluent will vary from kit to kit and is explicitly tested. Since standards are often prepared in analyte-free human serum, many protocols specify that the zero standard should be used to dilute high samples. If this is the case, enough zero should be provided for this purpose. When the method is to be used over a very wide range of concentrations and samples will frequently need dilution, the manufacturer should specify and supply the proper diluent. Even a specified diluent must be tested in actual use. On occasion a clinical sample must be diluted with a pool of normal serum or the patient's own baseline, or prestimulated, serum rather than the zero standard which has been chemically treated or lyophilized. Figure 5 illustrates examples of cases in which the selection of the best diluent significantly affected the accuracy of the final assay result.

E. Data Reduction

The selection of a method for handling standard curve data for routine use is a critical step in method evaluation and one which can have a profound effect on the user's ultimate satisfaction. Different data reduction methods have advantages and disadvantages related to their convenience of use, the rationality of the associated statistical inferences, the availability of needed computing power, and how well the mathematical model used corresponds to the actual biochemical reaction being monitored. Some antibodies in a particular assay simply do not react to give the simple, symmetric form assumed by the model. Thus, the real-

Table III. Diluents

1. Assay buffer containing protein
2. Zero standard—hormone-"free" serum
3. Stripped serum (charcoal, dextran coated charcoal)
4. Hypo-serum pool
5. Heterologous serum (horse, pig)
6. Simulated serum—albumin + TBG

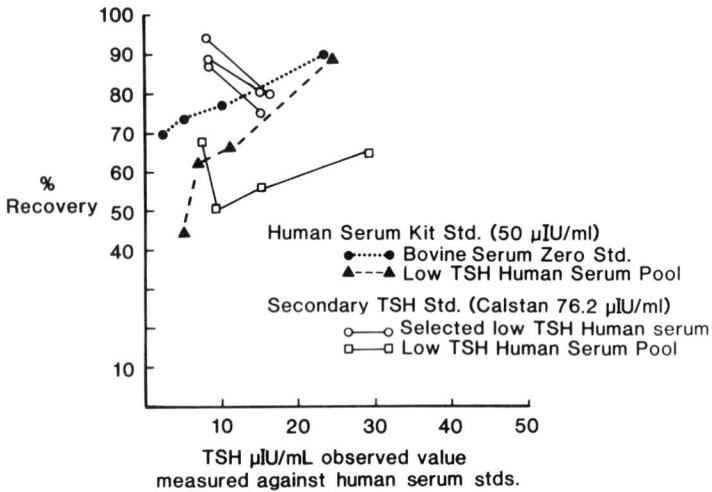

Figure 5. Effect of matrix on recovery of TSH. A high-TSH kit standard and a commercially available TSH (Calstan, Calbiochem) were diluted in the kit zero (●), a low-TSH serum pool (▲, □), or an individual patient sample (○). The recovery and parallelism varied with the diluent selected. Highest recovery was observed when a low-TSH serum from a single patient was used.

life standard curve may not be perfectly linearized in the logit–log plot, but may have another characteristic shape (Fig. 6). Some of this so-called "lack of fit" can be accounted for by poor precision and corrected by suitable weighting functions. Other assays will require an alternative model for accurate dose interpolation. Many calculators and computers used in immunoassay laboratories have available a selection of data reduction packages containing some index of the "goodness of fit." The extent to which actual standard points fit on the curve estabished by a given algorithm may be expressed quantitatively in various

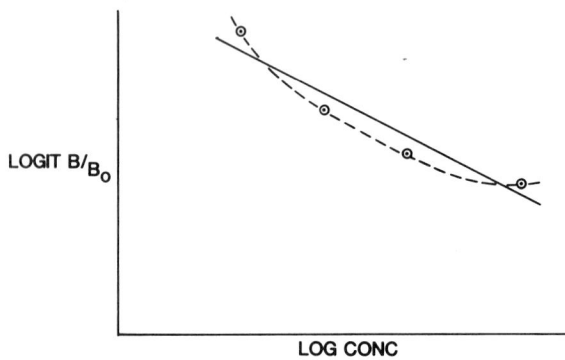

Figure 6. Typical standard curve not linearized by logit–log data reduction.

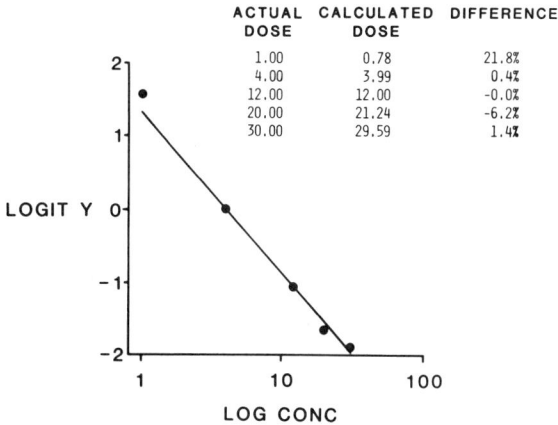

ACTUAL DOSE	CALCULATED DOSE	DIFFERENCE
1.00	0.78	21.8%
4.00	3.99	0.4%
12.00	12.00	-0.0%
20.00	21.24	-6.2%
30.00	29.59	1.4%

Figure 7. Typical standard curve not linearized by logit–log data reduction.

ways: percent deviation in dose units of the standard response from the best-fit line (Fig. 7), standard error of the estimate of the line, coefficient of linear correlation, or median variance ratio.

At initial evaluation, parameters of fit are noted and subsequent changes indicating a change of reagents or procedure which may adversely affect the performance of the kit are used for quality control. Often the fact that the points no longer fit the line well is the first indication that there has been some deterioration in a reagent.

VI. TRACER

A. Isotopic

In radioimmunoassay, the tracer is one of the most important contributors to assay performance and at the same time is the most variable. Aspects of performance attributed to poor tracer quality are decreased sensitivity, poor precision, increased nonspecific binding, overall decrease in binding, sudden drop in B_0, and loss of curve fit from lot to lot or with time. When such symptoms are observed, there is often very little the user can do to improve or investigate the situation other than replace the tracer and hope that a new lot and a new iodination will solve the problem.

A simplistic description of the immunologic reaction in a radioimmunoassay includes the implicit assumptions that all the tracer is labeled, can bind the antibody, can compete with the unlabeled antigen, and is present in trace quantities. In reality, the tracer may be unevenly labeled (different amount of iodine per molecule) or incompletely labeled (containing a substantial amount of un-labeled antigen).

In addition, the incorporation of iodine into proteins or haptens or the destructive effects of radioactive decay may alter the molecule such that it has a decreased ability to bind to the antibody or does not bind the antibody at all. Loss of immunoreactivity has the effect of increasing the apparent "free" fraction and altering the nonspecific binding characteristics independent of the reaction with antibody.

1. Specific Activity

Specific activity is the amount of radioactivity per unit of mass of ligand (Curies/mass). If tracers are produced in the laboratory, specific activity can be estimated by assuming that all of the protein added to the reaction mixture was iodinated and appears in the excluded peak after Sephadex chromatography. The radioactivity is assumed to be entirely distributed between the protein peak and the trailing iodine peak. Corrections for losses in the transfer and chromatography may be made if desired.

Specific activity of tracers can also be estimated by a technique called self-displacement (Fig. 8). Simply, the tracer is added to the radioimmunoassay reaction tube as if it were a sample. The mass of additional tracer added (not counting the usual aliquot which is incorporated in the estimation of zero) is read from a standard curve prepared with unlabeled standards. To increase the accuracy of the estimation of specific activity and tracer mass, several different

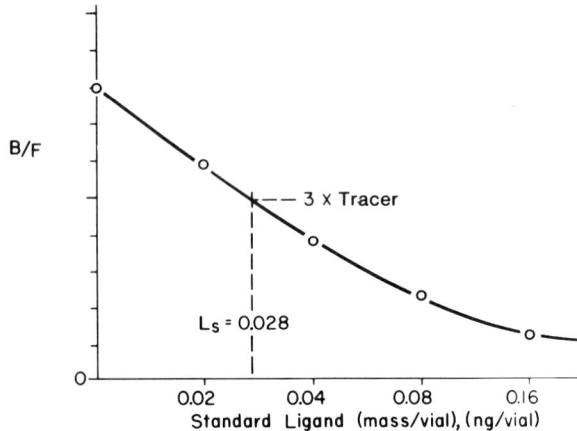

Figure 8. Specific activity by self-displacement. A standard curve is constructed (B/F vs. log dose). B/F is calculated for increments of tracer run as a sample. The figure illustrates that +3× tracer contains 0.028 ng. Thus the mass of tracer is 0.028/4 ng. Specific activity = TC(cpm or Ci)/0.007 ng.

aliquots of additional tracer are used, (e.g., $+1\times$, $+3\times$, $+10\times$). To be read from the standard curve, each sample response (B/F or B/T) is calculated individually, using the actual total counts in the aliquot corrected for the NSB tube containing the same increased amount of tracer. The mass of the tracer, corrected for sample size, should agree among the samples. If the response of tracer displacement is not parallel to the standard curve, the accuracy of the method may be affected (Englebienne and Slegers, 1983).

For the determination of specific activity, maximum slope in the low end of the standard curve is desirable, so the B/F versus dose plot is recommended. If desired, several statistical tests of the significance of the difference of slopes of the curves of labeled and unlabeled ligand may be made. Also, a t-test of the significance of differences of the masses observed with different sample sizes may demonstrate parallelism. For most routine evaluations, however, the more casual "eyeball" approach is adequate. Specific activity measured in this way is immunoreactive tracer since it is measured by its reaction with the specific antibody. Aside from being able to compare different methods with regard to the specific activity, and perhaps to infer relative assay sensitivity, the measured specific activity is used to calculate the total mass of tracer for the Scatchard plot (Sec. IX).

With some assay formats, the measurement of specific activity is impossible. If the tracer is prediluted, the additions may increase the reaction volume so much that the usual reaction kinetics, optimal reagent concentrations, and separation method are no longer similar to the original method. Occasionally a tracer will have such a high specific activity that no detectable displacement is seen. This is possible in the case of conjugate-labeled haptens.

2. Immunoreactivity

The ability of a tracer to bind to the antibody is called immunoreactivity. This property is measured by reacting a constant amount of tracer, usually the amount used in the assay, with increasing amounts of antibody until a plateau is reached. The maximum percent bound under these conditions is called the immunoreactive fraction (IF) (Fig. 9). Most calculations and theoretical models assume that all the tracer is immunoreactive. If the immunoreactivity is low ($<80\%$), then the assay may have poor sensitivity (F is too high and B/F is too low). Scatchard plots using labeled ligand will be nonlinear since both axes (B/F and B) depend on an accurate assessment of F or the total immunoreactive fraction. Better standard curves and Scatchard plots may be obtained by correcting the observed total counts (TC) for immunoreactive fraction (TC $\times$ IF) in all calculations. For example, $F_{corr} = B - (TC \times IF)$. Curves using B/B_0 should not be affected by IF unless the loss of immunoreactive tracer affects the chemical reaction itself. However, even if the standard curve is not affected, poor tracer quality may

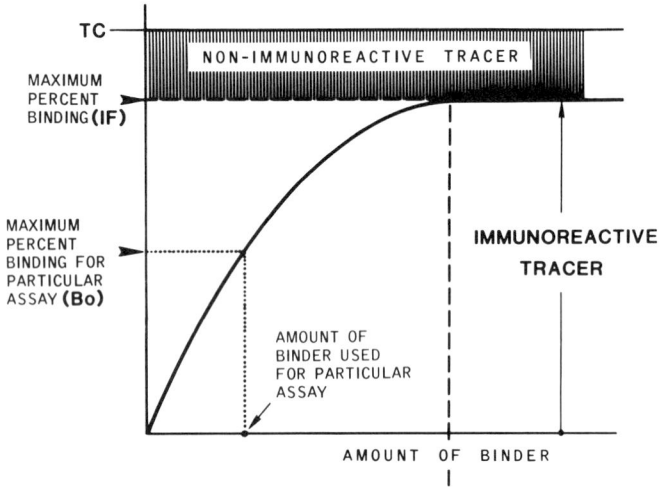

Figure 9. Immunoreactivity. Percent tracer bound (y axis) increases with increasing amount of binder (x axis) until a plateau is reached. The maximum binding as a percentage of total tracer is the immunoreactive fraction (IF).

mean differences between K and K^* ($K^* = K$ of the tracer), tracer lability, and unexpected cross-reactions.

B. Nonisotopic

Many of the tests used to evaluate tracer quality are related directly to the particular conditions and results of radioiodination. Specific activity measurement, for instance, is not easily translated to an equivalent test of enzyme- or fluorescence-labeled tracers. However, high immunoreactivity and low nonspecific binding should be expected for nonisotopic as well as isotopic tracers. Tests for these properties are the same as those previously described. In addition, each tracer should be carefully reviewed for the presence of any unique instability, inadequate optimization, or any special interferences which might be related to the biochemical characteristics of the tracer itself.

VII. SENSITIVITY

Sensitivity, the smallest amount of measurable ligand that is reliably not zero, is a characteristic of the standard curve and reflects the affinity of the antibody, the specific activity (low mass) of the tracer, and the suitability of the blank. This characteristic of the assay is relatively easy to understand conceptually but is somewhat more complex in analytical terms. Sensitivity depends on both the slope of the standard curve and the precision of individual measurements at or near zero. For two assays with the same precision at zero, the steepest curve is the most sensitive, that is, has the greatest change in measurable response per small change in dose. For two assays with the same slope, the more precise is the more sensitive (Fig. 10).

The least detectable dose (LDD), commonly used to define sensitivity, is measured by assaying replicates of the zero standard (e.g., 10 replicates) and calculating the mean counts bound and standard deviation. The mean is used for the standard curve, and the response, mean cpm $-$ 2 SD, read in dose or mass from the standard curve is the LDD, that is, the smallest dose that is not zero with 95% confidence. However, since the zero standard is often a modified sample (treated serum, buffer, etc.), the precision of this measurement may be greater than that of a patient sample. If the LDD is much less than the lowest standard it is often desirable to prepare a standard curve with additional standards in the low end. This curve demonstrates the linearity and precision of the curve in that range. As with the specific activity measurement, a B/F plot with its steep slope in the low end is recommended in order to get an accurate measure of LDD. It is a very practical problem to decide whether to report results between the lowest standard and the LDD. Common sense and a careful evaluation of the shape of the curve, the measured LDD, and clinical need all contribute to the answer.

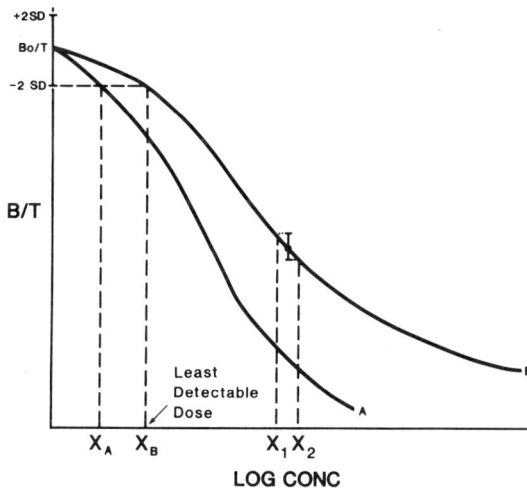

Figure 10. Least detectable dose (LDD). The precision of B_0 is calculated on replicates. The dose level corresponding to $B_0 - 2$ SD is the LDD (X_A, X_B). $X_2 - X_1$ is the "resolution," or minimal difference in dose distinguishable.

Table IV. How to Improve Sensitivity

---

1. Increase sample size. Be sure to test the effect of matrix and volume changes.
2. Dilute antibody (competitive assay). Dilutions will shift the curve down and to the left, affecting the total binding, precision, and range, as well as slope.
3. Increase reaction time or temperature. This may affect the low end of the curve more than the high end.
4. Add tracer sequentially. This will increase the slope and also increase the number of steps and reduce precision.
5. For IRMA, increase antibody, time, or sample size.

The same argument can be made for any point on the standard curve. Each point is associated with a measurement error (mean response ± 2 SD). The term "resolution" is used to describe the smallest difference in dose that can be distinguished from another. Just as when we consider the curve near zero, the resolution depends on both precision and slope.

If the sensitivity of a method is less than desired, it is possible to modify the assay according to well-known principles. Any modified assay must, of course, be as thoroughly evaluated and optimized as the original before it can be used routinely. Tests of sensitivity as well as specificity must be repeated for any modification of the assay protocol. Manufacturers' claims and guarantees are valid only for the protocol that was approved and sold. Even if no modifications are made, it may be useful to review the experimental variables that contribute to sensitivity. Table IV lists a variety of measures which can be predicted to increase sensitivity. Testing some of these at the time of assay evaluation will demonstrate how robust the assay is to small changes in reaction conditions.

VIII. EVALUATION OF ACCURACY

Accuracy is a complex concept which reflects the ability of the assay to measure the true value of analyte. An accurate test is implicitly both specific and precise. Accuracy can be affected by every component of the immunoassay: systematic errors (cross-reactivity or poor recovery), poor tracer, lack of specificity of the antibody, and poor precision (technical errors, low-affinity antibody, or poor-quality tracer). Although difficult to define simply, and impossible to prove in a single test, it is easy to describe the characteristics of an accurate immunoassay.

A. Standards

All expectations of an accurate chemical measurement rest fundamentally on the concept of standardization and the characteristics of the standard itself. An ideal standard has the following characteristics: (1) the analyte is chemically well defined, homogeneous, and available in pure form, and (2) the standard is immunologically identical to the analyte of interest in a universally valid matrix. Unfortunately, for many of the analytes measured by radioimmunoassay, almost none of these is true. Some protein hormones are not completely characterized; others exist in a variety of forms including pre- and prohormones, hormone fragments, and forms varying in carbohydrate content. International standards and reference preparations are often mixtures of proteins which are defined in terms of biological activity and may differ chemically depending on the source or matrix (serum, urine, tissue extract). Other analytes such as drugs and vitamins are well characterized chemically and are available in pure form. Still, ultimate accuracy depends on a pure standard. For specificity, the antibody should react only with the analyte of interest in a well-defined sample, and the reaction should be free of significant nonspecific interferences.

Although no single laboratory test can prove accuracy, several tests may be done which address different aspects of the complex situation. Failure to perform well in one of these experimental tests may disprove accuracy or at least raise questions regarding the validity of the assay.

B. Parallelism

An essential validation of test accuracy is the so-called test of parallelism. It answers the frequently encountered question, "If I dilute a patient sample, will I get the same answer, corrected for the dilution? If I don't, which is the 'right' answer?" Alternative ways to pose this problem are, "Is the assayed value independent of the sample size?" and "Do dilutions of the unknown parallel the standard curve?" Surely if the answer to these questions is "No" then the test cannot be accurate.

Parallelism on dilution is demonstrated by diluting a sample or standard with an appropriate diluent and running the assay. Several different patient samples should be tested, including at least three different dilutions per sample to demonstrate linearity. Dilutions should be selected so that they fall within the linear and most precise portion of the standard curve. Results of the experiment can be displayed in several different ways in order to evaluate parallelism. One of the simplest methods is to calculate the final concentration by multiplying by the appropriate dilution and plot the result against dilution or sample size (Fig. 11). A parallel response is inferred from a horizontal line. It is possible to apply statistical tests for the significance of the difference of the slope from zero or a t-test of the significance of the difference of one dilution from another. However, visual inspection is usually adequate for a good sense of the performance of a method. A plot of observed value (not corrected for dilution) versus dilution should be linear. Observed versus expected (based on the undiluted value) should

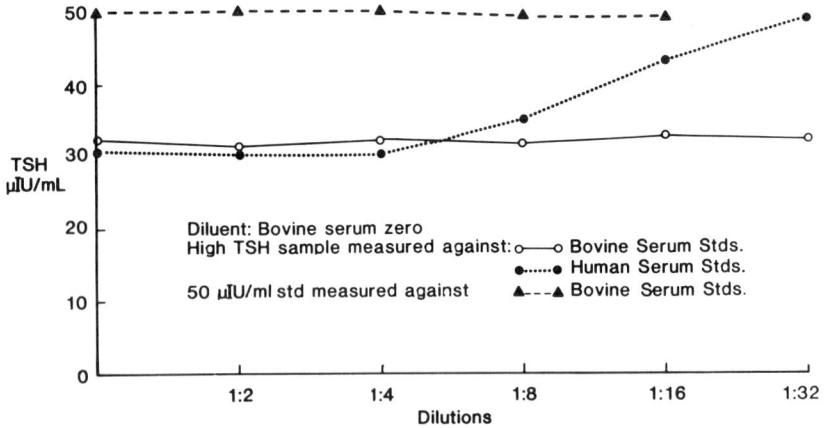

Figure 11. Parallelism. A high-TSH patient sample (○, ●) and a kit standard, 50 μIU/ml TSH (▲), were diluted in the kit zero standard containing bovine serum. Dilutions were parallel when compared with standards containing bovine serum but not parallel compared with standards containing human serum. The nonparallel response appeared to be related to the changing matrix in the diluted sample relative to the standard curve.

be a 45° line. Different samples displayed together should be parallel to each other. If the intercept is not zero, the assay may show parallelism but also a bias.

1. Diluents

Selection of the appropriate diluent is essential. The diluent must be of a matrix similar enough to the sample that the changing matrix in the diluted sample does not in itself cause loss of parallelism. Even the zero standard which is often recommended may result in a matrix that varies enough that it is detected as nonparallelism.

In addition to diluting several patient samples, dilute the highest kit standard with the diluent of choice. The diluted standards should be parallel to the standard curve if the diluent is compatible. Occasionally a nonparallel response has revealed that the kit standards were not all from the same source or that the assigned standard values were not based on dilutions of an independently assayed mass, but had been adjusted to fit a preset curve or previous quality control values. These adjustments by the manufacturer are invisible to the user of a kit and make it very difficult to solve problems and interpret patient results in the routine laboratory.

A final experimental consideration for performing tests of parallelism is the ever-important blank. Since the NSB tube was optimized to correct for non-specific effects under standard (undiluted) conditions, it is not necessarily appropriate for application to diluted samples.

2. *Causes of Nonparallelism*

When dilutions of patient samples do not agree, the effect may be due to an experimental error: improper diluent, improper blanking, poor selection of dilution, or dilution error.

Fundamental characteristics of the antigen–antibody reaction may also cause nonparallelism. For example, if the antigen is present in a variety of chemical forms, reaction with antibody may not be identical to that of the standard. Antibody heterogeneity in polyclonal antisera may result in nonparallelism. Figure 12 shows lack of agreement with a simple 1 : 2 dilution of patient samples in a ferritin RIA. This effect was apparent at concentrations greater than 200 ng/ml and was attributed to antibody heterogeneity, later confirmed by a nonlinear Scatchard plot.

Although the antigen is expected to react linearly on dilution, interfering substances usually do not. Lack of agreement on dilution was one of the early symptoms of the effects of endogenous insulin antibodies in the serum of patients taking insulin. Perlstein (1978; Perlstein *et al.*, 1980) used tests of parallelism to show the effect of drugs and other interfering substances on accuracy.

C. Recovery

The test most often used in the clinical chemical literature to demonstrate the accuracy of an assay is a recovery study. The objective of a recovery study is to

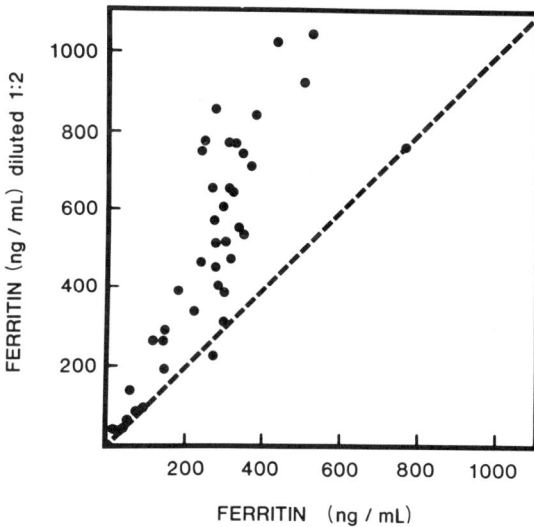

Figure 12. Parallelism. The graph shows patient samples assayed in a ferritin RIA undiluted (*x* axis) and diluted 1 : 2 with the kit zero standard (*y* axis). Good agreement was observed below 200 ng/ml.

Table V. Recovery Study

---
1. Prepare and analyze ''base''
2. Obtain purified analyte
3. Choose appropriate concentrations of analyte and base
4. Measure base plus analyte
5. Calculate recovery
---

test whether a known increment of analyte added to a sample can be measured quantitatively by the assay being examined. Although some types of systematic error (proportional matrix effect) are demonstrated, a recovery will not detect others. Thus, it is a good test in the negative, but a positive test still does not prove that an assay is accurate. Recoveries are often cited in the research literature and in kit brochures, but they are not frequently done in routine clinical laboratories because they are relatively expensive and are difficult to do well. Also, a variety of technical problems make the results difficult to interpret. Table V summarizes the steps of the experimental protocol.

1. Experimental Steps

The first step is to obtain pure, assayed, stable standard material. This is possible for some analytes: pure chemicals such as drugs, vitamins, steroid and small peptide hormones, and thyroid hormones. International standards are available for a few peptide hormones, but these are not necessarily pure and are assigned values based on activity. Kit standards and standards from other kits are often the only materials conveniently available. These are not truly appropriate, since the assay is already standardized with them. Differences in standard matrix between kits occasionally preclude even this simple cross-check.

The ''spike'' or added standard is prepared as accurately as possible, using an analytical balance and volumetric glassware. The prepared sample should be in high enough concentration that the addition does not significantly dilute the matrix. Some analytes, for example, tetrahydrofolic acid, are highly sensitive to oxidative conditions and pH. The amount of spike added should be large enough to be detected precisely.

Selection of the base material (sample) to which the spike is added is critical. The concentration of the base is measured (in the same assay) and is assumed to be accurate. Unfortunately, this is exactly the point we are trying to prove. For this reason, and to reduce the absolute effect of any errors in the base measurement, a base which contains little or none of the analyte of interest is selected whenever possible. Both the base material and the base containing the spike are measured in the assay being tested.

2. Calculation

When the base alone and the base plus the spike are measured, recovery (R) can be calculated in two ways. When the assay is accurate, both methods of calculation will give $R = 100\%$. If the assay is not accurate, the calculations will differ. Method 1 will give a maximum estimate of a proportional or matrix error. Using method 2, it is not possible to make any inference regarding the nature of the error. Neither will detect a constant error in the base as well as the measurement including the spike.

$$?$$
$$\text{Recovery standard } (A) + \text{base } (B) = \text{analyte observed } (C)$$

Method 1: $R =$ (amt. observed $-$ amt. in base)/amt. added $\times$ 100. $R(\%) = (C - B)/A \times 100$. This method assumes that A is known exactly and attributes all lack of accuracy to loss of the added spike. Method 1 gives the lowest (least favorable) R. However, if R, for example, were 50%, a proportional error (effect of matrix) could be inferred. Then we must also conclude that there was a 50% error in the original base measurement (B) as well.

Method 2: $R =$ (amt. observed/amt. expected) $\times$ 100, where amt. expected = amt. in base + amt. added. $R(\%) = C/(A + B) \times 100$. This is the most common calculation and yields the greater R, if $R < 100\%$. When R = 100% by this calculation, no inference about the error in the base can be made.

Before extreme joy or despair is experienced over the outcome of a recovery experiment, some thought should be given to what are to be the acceptable limits of the study. Calculation by either method requires three measurements by assays with known precision in the ranges used. Errors propagated through the equation will give the expected error in R.

D. Cross-Reactivity

Specificity is the ability of an assay to produce a measurable response only for the analyte of interest. For immunoassays this property is the result of the inherent nature of the immune system, which can produce an almost limitless variety of binding sites on immunoglobulins which have a very strong affinity for specific chemical structures on antigens. Since antigenic determinants may be shared or are similar among classes of molecules, cross-reactivity, or overlap in binding specificity, is common. In practical terms, does the antibody react with any other substances likely to be found in any sample analyzed? Cross-reactivity data are often published. However, it may be desirable to test some compounds in the laboratory to verify the accuracy with current lots of reagent and to test additional substances when applicable. Usually this is done very selectively

$$\text{Cross reactivity at 50\% displacement} = \frac{\text{mass of standard}}{\text{mass of competitor}} \times 100$$

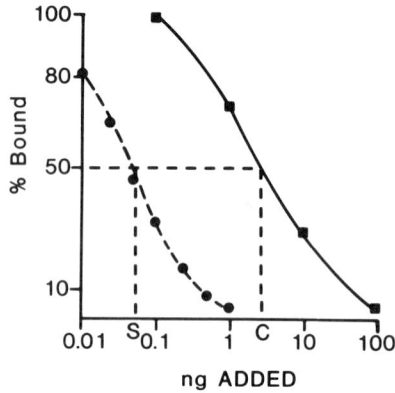

Figure 13. Cross-reactivity. A displacement curve for a cross-reacting substance (■) is compared to the standard curve (●). The dose at 50% displacement, *S*, divided by the dose of competitor, *C*, is the fractional cross-reactivity in mass units.

when specific problems can be anticipated or to answer a specific question. An example of a useful test of cross-reactivity performed during an evaluation in our laboratory was a test of luteinizing hormone (LH) reactivity in β-HCG kit. Initial studies had demonstrated a cross-reactivity of 4%. Later, during routine use when quality control (QC) shifts were observed, retesting showed 10% cross-reactivity of LH, which accounted for the shifts and also the inaccuracy observed in patient samples.

1. Calculation

Cross-reactivity is usually expressed as the relative dose required to displace 50% of the maximum tracer binding (Fig. 13). The experiment is done by running an entire standard curve of the cross-reacting substance as well as the usual standard curve. Cross-reactivity = (mass of standard at 50% B_0)/(mass of competitor at 50% B_0) × 100. Even when the apparent cross-reactivity is acceptably low, it is important to pay attention to the concentrations of possible interfering substances in samples being measured.

The displacement curve of cross-reacting substances is often not parallel to that of the standard ligand. This means that the interference will not be the same at all concentrations of the unknown. Clearly, reported cross-reactivities are meant to give only a general idea of possible inaccuracy due to lack of specificity of the antibody.

IX. ANTIBODY CHARACTERISTICS

Specificity of an immunoassay is determined by the unique biosynthesis of antibodies and the role they play in the capability of the immune system to identify foreign antigens (Edelman, 1973; Tonegawa et al., 1974; Seidman et al., 1978). Sensitivity of an assay is determined primarily by the characteristic antibody affinity constant (K) and the antibody titer in the assay (Zettner, 1973; Walker and Kean, 1977). Evaluation of antisera usually includes measurement of the average affinity constant (K) by Scatchard analysis. Under ideal conditions, a linear relationship between the ratio of bound to free ligand (B/F) and the mass of the bound ligand (B) will result (Fig. 14). The slope of this linear graph is the negative of the affinity constant (K) characteristic of the ligand for the antibody; if the relationship is not linear, at best the slope of the plot yields a mean or an "average" affinity (see Chapter 1). Frequently observed nonlinear shapes (Fig. 14) have been attributed to multiple populations of antibodies, nonspecific binding, negative cooperativity, or inequality of the affinities of the labeled (K^*) and nonlabeled (K) ligand for the antibody (Rodbard et al., 1971; Feldman et al., 1972; Hollemans and Bertina, 1975; Bremner and Chase, 1980).

A. Monitoring Component Stability

Effective and appropriate use of an assay requires an appreciation of its limitations. As with any assay, two important limitations of immunoassays are specificity and sensitivity. These limitations are strongly influenced by, but not limited to, the properties of the antibody. Specificity of an RIA is determined by the antibody amino acid sequence, the structure of the ligand, and the composition of the incubation matrix. Sensitivity of an assay is determined by the affinity

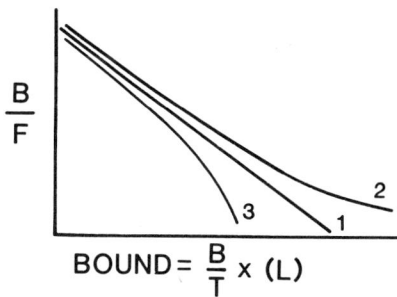

Figure 14. Scatchard plot. B/F counts (y axis) are plotted against bound mass. When all assumptions are met, the curve is linear (Bernutz et al., 1985). Scatchard plots may also be nonlinear (Bremner and Chase, 1980; Chervu and Murty, 1975). For RIA, bound mass is estimated from B/T (cpm) $\times$ L (total ligand mass).

of the antibody for the ligand, the antibody concentration, and the amount of tracer in the reaction mixture (Feldman *et al.*, 1972; Chervu and Murty, 1975; Yallow, 1980; Fernandez *et al.*, 1983).

The stability of assay sensitivity for a defined set of reaction conditions can readily be monitored. This can be accomplished by logging an intercept point such as the dose at 80% or 90% displacement (ED_{80} or ED_{90}) or the dose at some multiple of the B_0 standard deviation from the B_0 (Rodbard *et al.*, 1968).

The stability of the specificity of the assay system, however, is much more difficult to monitor. Maintaining specificity of an assay system depends on the stability of each major reagent—tracer, calibration standard, and binder reagent (antiserum or monoclonal antibody)—and the extent of homogeneity of each reagent. If each reagent behaved as if it contained a single population of molecular species, the assay specificity would depend on the extent to which other compounds competed with the tracer and ligand of interest for the same binding sites. With nonhomogeneous reagents, however, the relative concentrations and affinities of "contaminating" molecular species can change assay specificity. Lack of ideal specificity may be tolerable in an assay as long as it is recognized, is understood in terms of potential physiological levels, and does not change significantly over the working range of the assay, either as reagents age in storage or as different lots are used.

There is considerable likelihood that, with time, the tracer will change in composition in both labeled and nonlabeled molecular species. These changes can be due to ordinary chemical instability, to so-called decay catastrophe, or to both. The purity of the calibration standards can also deteriorate over time due to ordinary chemical instabilities and the storage conditions. Antibodies (or antisera) are generally more stable than either the tracer or the standards. A calculation based on Scatchard analysis using standard curve data can provide insight on whether aging reagents might modify assay specificity.

B. Assay-Conditional Scatchard Plot

1. Calculation

Calculation of the parameters (B/F and bound ligand mass) required for a Scatchard plot is easily done from RIA data. Derivation of binding affinity or binding sites, however, may be inappropriate because assays are often not performed under conditions that allow compliance with critical assumptions underlying the rigorous Scatchard plot. Lack of compliance with these assumptions can cause the graph to deviate from the theoretically linear form for a variety of reasons. Although the curve may be nonlinear, a reproducible nonlinear shape can provide insight into the stability of assay reagents. Many assay systems have a stable graph shape over the storage life of the reagents. This stability provides presumptive evidence about reagent stability. The simplicity of calculating B/F and bound ligand mass (B) makes this qualitative use of the Scatchard plot readily available to any laboratory. To emphasize that the use to which the Scatchard plot is being put in this RIA context is qualitative, we will refer to the plot generated from RIA standard curve data as an assay-conditional Scatchard plot (ACSP).

Calculation of the graph parameters, B/F and B, can be accomplished by either of two approaches, one using minimal corrections, the other using nonspecific binding corrections (Dotti and Castagnetti, 1978):

METHOD 1

Bound-to-free ratio (B/F):

$$\frac{\text{net bound tracer (counts)}}{\text{net free tracer (counts)}}$$

Bound ligand (B):

$$\frac{\text{net bound tracer (counts)}}{\text{net total tracer (counts)}} \times \text{total ligand mass (cold + tracer)}$$

METHOD 2

Bound-to-free ratio (B/F):

$$\frac{C_b - \text{NSB}}{T - (C_b - \text{NSB})}$$

Bound ligand (B):

$$(L_s + L_t) \times C_b/T$$

where C_b is net bound counts; T, net total counts; NSB, net nonspecific binding counts; L_s, ligand in reaction volume contributed from standard; and L_t, ligand in reaction volume contributed from tracer (can be estimated from manufacturer's information or from a "self-displacement" assay).

2. Interpretation

In rigorous Scatchard analysis, the expected graphical representation of B/F and B will be a straight line (Scatchard, 1949). Underlying this theoretical graph, however, are specific assumptions that must be categorically true for this expected linear form to occur (Smith and Feldkamp, 1979). These assumptions include (a) first-order mass action kinetics, (b) homogeneous reagents, (c) thermodynamic equilibrium, and (d) an unbiased measure of bound and free ligand in the presence of the binder and reaction matrix. These requirements translate to the immunoassay as follows: (a) while the antiserum may in fact be multivalent, the binding sites must not demonstrate strong cooperativity, (b) the antiserum reagent, the labeled ligand, and the nonlabeled ligand must each behave as if it were homogeneous throughout the assay range, (c) the assay reaction must be indistinguishable from equilibrium. The assumption of an unbiased measure of the distribution of free and bound ligand requires that the binding affinities of the labeled and nonlabeled ligands be essentially equivalent over the range of the assay, that the separation of bound and free ligand be 100% efficient, and that the separation procedure not disrupt the primary antigen–antibody complex.

Attention must also be directed to the meaning of the numerical quantities used in the above equations. Even if all assumptions on the underlying reactions are met, the numbers used in the equations may not have their presumed or intended meaning. As a result, curvature can be introduced in the plot by numerical artifact rather than the underlying chemistry (Smith, 1985). For example, T will overestimate the total amount of labeled ligand if the tracer immunoreactive fraction is significantly less than 100% because the assumption of isotope dilution will be invalid. Some correction of the counts bound for nonspecific or background binding is required. The quantity L_t may be unavailable to a kit user or, if it is measured by the tracer displacement method described above, may be subject to measurement bias. Nonspecific binding is the easiest of these quantities to approximate routinely (Sec. V,C,3).

Using an estimate for NSB, each tube of bound labeled ligand can be corrected by subtracting NSB, the count level in the appropriately determined nonspecific binding tube. Correct determination of NSB, however, also depends on the validity of the fundamental assumptions for tracer dilution analysis, that is, 100% immunoreactivity and equal affinity of cold and labeled ligand for the "nonspecific" binding sites. The coordinates for the ACSP using this correction are calculated by method 2.

Table VI. Causes of Nonlinear Scatchard Plots

---

1. Concave at high ligand concentration:
   Nonequilibrium; K^*/K decreases over the assay range or $K^*/K > 1$ even if the ratio is constant over the assay range; the separation efficiency of bound and free is significantly less than 100%; the separation process disrupts the antigen–antibody complex; NSB is overestimated; or the immunoreactive fraction is less than 100%
2. Convex at high ligand concentration:
   Multiple binding sites; K^*/K increases over the assay range or $K^*/K > 1$ even if the ratio is constant over the assay range; NSB is underestimated; or there is negative cooperativity
3. Concave at low ligand concentrations:
   Positive cooperativity; tracer mass is underestimated; or the immunoreactive fraction is less than 100%
4. Convex at low ligand concentration:
   Multiple binding sites; or overestimated tracer mass

Assay-conditional Scatchard plots constructed using either method 1 or method 2 are generally not linear. The nonlinear curves can be grouped according to shape. Curves may be concave or convex at high ligand concentrations and/or concave or convex at low ligand concentrations. By theoretical considerations alone, a violation of each of the fundamental assumptions described above can be associated with a nonlinear shape generated by the effect on the underlying reaction or calculation (Table VI, Fig. 15). A linear ACSP indicates that an assay system may have functionally homogeneous binder, calibrator, and tracer, that $K^* = K$ over the assay range, and that the estimate of the tracer mass used was

Reaction condition	Deviation from linearity	
I. Positive cooperativity	Low-dose hook	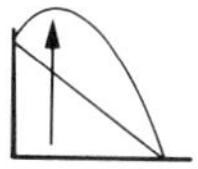
II. Negative cooperativity	Right skew	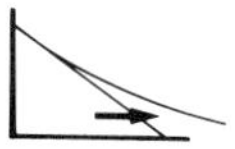
III. Multiple binding sites	Right skew	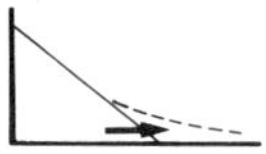
IV. Affinity for binder A. Affinity of labeled ligand is greater than that of the calibration ligand	Right skew	
B. Affinity of calibration ligand is greater than that of the labeled ligand	Left skew	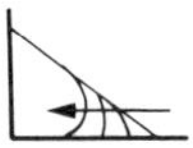
V. Nonequilibrium reaction	Left skew	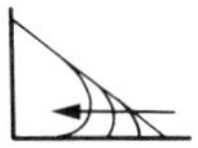
VI. Separation efficiency of bound from free is significantly less than 100%.	Left skew	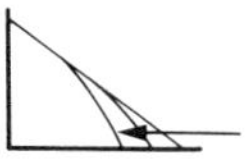
VII. Separation disrupts the ligand–binder complex.	Left skew	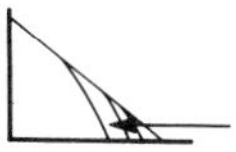

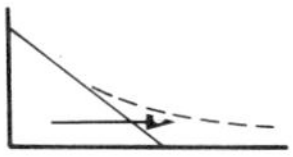

Figure 15. Reaction conditions that may result in nonlinear Scatchard plots. A variety of reaction conditions are shown with an illustration of how the Scatchard plot can be affected. Note that the left skew due either to poor separation efficiency (VI) or to disruption of the complex (VII) cannot "curl" back on itself as can the left skew due either to different affinity constants (IV,B) or to lack of equilibrium (V).

reasonably accurate. A linear ACSP, however, may also represent a fortuitous balance of opposing influences on the curve shape.

Although some of the relationships among the immunoassay components may account for lack of parallelism and/or specificity, others will have little or no effect. Any one or a combination of the following violations of the fundamental assumptions may cause variable parallelism and/or specificity within the assay range: positive or negative cooperativity, multiple binding sites, or variable K^*/K ratio either within the assay range or between assays. Some will mask the impact of others or can be masked by violations that have little or no effect on assay parallelism and/or specificity. For example, the impact of negative cooperativity, secondary binding sites, or an increasing K^*/K ratio may be masked by one or more of the following: (a) nonequilibrium conditions, (b) poor separation of bound and free tracer, (c) a separation process that significantly disrupts the antigen–antibody complex, (d) overestimation of the NSB, or (e) a low immunoreactive fraction. The impact of decreasing K^*/K ratio over the assay range on the ACSP shape may be masked by (a) an underestimated NSB, (b) negative cooperativity, and/or (c) multiple binding sites.

Although a variety of shapes are possible, a particular assay system run with constant conditions will have a characteristic ACSP shape resulting from a balance among the various influences on the theoretical form. This "characteristic ACSP" is observed from run to run except for minor statistical variations. When the underlying chemistry of a reagent changes or a variation in temperature or timing occurs, the ACSP may also change. The ACSP can thus serve as an indicator to alert the laboratorian to a chemical instability in one or more of the reagents in an assay. Since a variable ACSP is a symptom of a changing K^*/K ratio over the assay range, a consistent ACSP shape is desirable from run to run. Operating from the position that a stable shape is more important than a particular shape, time and effort should be concentrated on assays or assay conditions that have a consistent ACSP shape and, therefore, a better chance of having uniform specificity and/or parallelism. Variations of this sort observed in Scatchard plots may be due to the preparation and optimization of the reagents themselves or to poorly controlled shipping or storage conditions. The overall utility of the ACSP as a tool is that, without extra costs, the laboratorian can be alerted to assays that are sensitive to conditions that may compromise the quality of the assay.

A frequently observed modification of ACSP shape as reagents age is a shift toward the left with the high concentration end being more affected than the low end (left skew) (Fig. 16). Based on the correlation between the curve shapes and the underlying chemistry discussed above, we can infer which components of the assay are most likely to change over time. Among those discussed, the most likely to be stable over time are (a) the degree to which equilibrium is reached in the assay (assuming constant incubation time and temperature), (b) separation

Numerical error	Shape artifact
I. NSB A. Too large	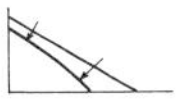
B. Too small	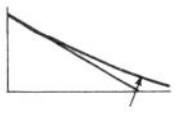
II. Tracer mass A. Underestimated	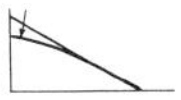
B. Overestimated	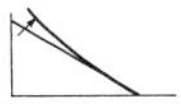
III. Immunoreactivity $<100\%$	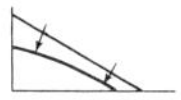

Figure 16. Effects of incorrect numerical estimates on the shape of the Scatchard plot. Nonspecific binding, tracer mass, and tracer immunoreactivity are three constants used to calculate the Scatchard plot parameters that may be difficult to estimate accurately. Qualitative effects on the overall shape of the Scatchard plot due to inaccurate estimates of these constants are illustrated.

efficiency, and (c) the degree to which the antigen–antibody complex is disrupted by the separation process. The remaining assumptions related to this shape may not hold as reagents age or as reagent lots change: (a) K^* may decrease relative to K, (b) NSB may increase, or (c) the immunoreactive fraction may decrease. Each of these changes can be related to the effects of time, storage, or decay on the tracer. If tracer deterioration primarily affects K^*, the shape of the low concentration end of the curve will remain relatively unchanged. If, however, a decrease in the tracer immunoreactive fraction and/or the tracer immunoreactive mass is significant, the low ligand end of the ACSP will become concave as well.

It is important to recognize that a linear shape may or may not be preferable to a consistent nonlinear shape. For example, a nonequilibrium assay may have good parallelism and specificity even though its ACSP is nonlinear. Also, an assay with K^* not equal to K (but K^*/K constant within the assay range) may have uniform parallelism and good specificity even though the ACSP is nonlinear.

The ACSP can be used as a quality control tool with routine assays. When the characteristic ACSP is known, it may be used to spot-check or to routinely follow assay performance. An abrupt change in the ACSP shape may signal a significant change in the character of a reagent, a change in reagent storage conditions, or poor adherence to the assay protocol, and may reflect current or future problems with the assay.

X. MONITORING REACTION CONDITIONS

Although a method may perform well in initial evaluation runs, the performance under expected laboratory running conditions should be tested. For a fair test, the manufacturer's recommended time and temperature conditions must be followed to the letter. If, for convenience in the laboratory, incubation times are shortened or lengthened, or reagents are combined before additions, the user must validate any such changes. The kit should be tested with full-sized runs to check for front-to-back drift. The "robustness" of an assay to environmental changes will profoundly affect long-term satisfaction with a particular kit. If drift or imprecision is a problem, limiting the run size or perhaps timing individual racks separately may be required for the assay to be reliable.

XI. CLINICAL VALIDATION

The final step is the most critical to a clinical laboratory's customer, the physician. The physician is most interested in whether the result is clinically meaningful. Sometimes, especially with a new test, the value remains to be established. Other new tests appear to have the potential to answer burning clinical questions (e.g., free T_4 or prostatic acid phosphatase), but we are disappointed because the state of our knowledge of physiology or disease is incomplete. The best assay can measure only what is present. If an analyte is not reliably associated with the disease process, even the perfect assay will fail in its purpose.

A. Patient Samples

Although some patient specimens are run at early stages of evaluation, usually an extensive testing or validation of the assay with clinical samples is delayed until a method has been tentatively selected. Although the manufacturer, supplementing the medical literature, will have established the expected values in certain diseases, the laboratory should verify the claims by running samples from patients with known disease. A method is expected to reflect hyper- or hypofunction consistent with clinical and other biochemical parameters and to show appropriate changes after the patient is treated or when suppression or stimulation tests are done. A change in method sensitivity or specificity can be very important, as stimulation tests are often interpreted on the basis of increase over baseline values.

Enhanced discrimination between normal and abnormal is usually the primary objective of new laboratory tests. For some diseases, overlap is inherent in the physiology. However, the TSH experience serves to illustrate that improved assay sensitivity and specificity can contribute to such discrimination. Studies by Seth *et al.* (1984) and by Bernutz *et al.* (1985) demonstrate that with use of monoclonal antibodies and IRMA technology, along with sensitive detection techniques, hyperthyroid (i.e., low TSH) can be distinguished from euthyroid patients and that the patients with lowest TSH have a flat response to thyrotropin-releasing hormone (TRH). This application is a marked change from a few years ago, when the normal range overlapped zero.

When a test is new or difficult to interpret, a follow-up on abnormal results by consulting with a clinician or by reviewing the patient record should confirm that the test is giving clinically meaningful results. Although extensive review of this type may be beyond the scope of many laboratories, this information will enhance confidence in a new assay.

B. Comparison with Reference Methods

A common way to establish some confidence in the clinical validity is to split samples between the new method and an assay currently in use, a commercial laboratory, or a reference method. A graph of the two methods plotted against one another demonstrates general correspondence between methods by visual inspection. Correlation and linear regression and other statistical methods of comparison are available. Concordance between methods (agreement in the number of normals and abnormals) can be calculated. However, simple visualization of points appearing in the quadrants separated by the normal ranges of each method is often sufficient to identify significant discrepancies. To establish clinical validity of a new method it may be necessary to investigate individual discrepancies and identify the cause. Occasionally the discrepancy can be explained by an analytical error or an interference influencing one method but not the other. In the example of prostatic acid phosphatase (Fig. 17), some apparently high values in the absence of disease (and in some women) could be attributed to the effects of lipemia on the assay. Evaluation of concordance depends, of course, on the limits of normal used on the graph. If a laboratory normal range is actually lower or higher than the manufacturer's, that range should be used in order to avoid misclassification. Another consideration in interpreting the graph is the sensitivity of each assay. If one is much more sensitive than another, values will be spread out on one axis, contributing to a nonlinear relationship and poor correlation.

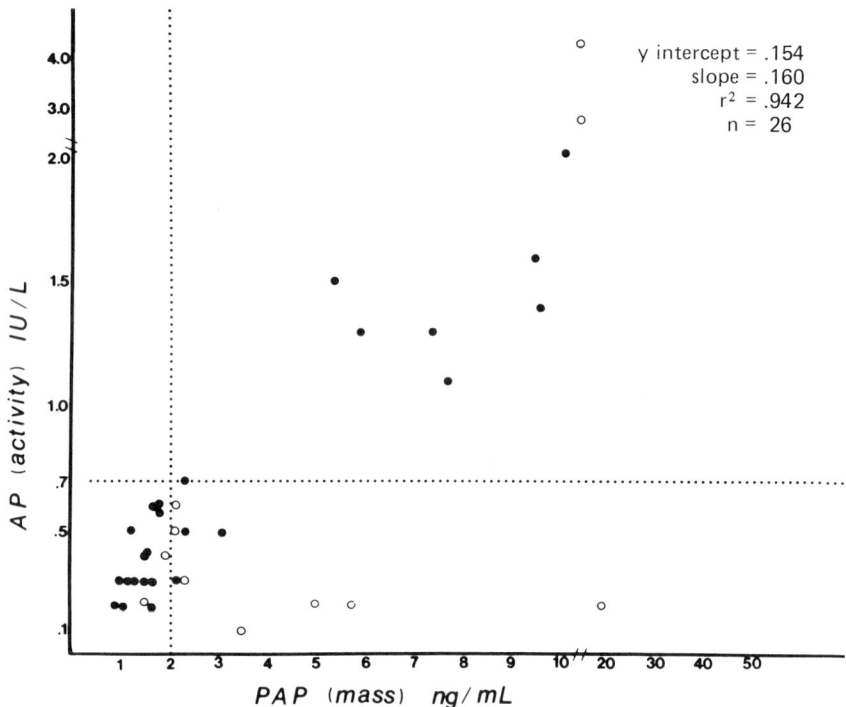

Figure 17. Split sample comparison. An RIA for prostatic acid phosphatase (PAP) was compared with an enzymatic method (Dupont ACA). Normal ranges for each method are denoted by dotted lines. Patient samples (some lipemic) not included in the calculations are denoted by (O).

C. Normal Range

The concept of normal range and the practical problems associated with the determination of normal, or reference, ranges for clinical laboratory tests are knotty problems for the laboratory. Unfortunately, even when the laboratory buys kits already optimized and ready to use, the requirement to address normal range determination is not solved. Intellectually, it is easy to appreciate that for any test to be interpretable there must be some comparison with what is expected. For the comparison to be clinically useful, the reference population must be an adequate representation of the patient population, but without disease. Elaborate semantic and philosophical arguments have revolved around whether normal ranges are necessarily "healthy" or "optimal" ranges.

Normal ranges are generally described in the medical literature when a test or a new technology is introduced. Since sensitivity and specificity are often technique-dependent, ranges described in the literature may or may not be achievable in a routine laboratory. An example of how the normal range changes with methodology is TSH immunoassay. Although research assays (with long incubation times) originally described normal ranges of <5 mIU/liter, kit assays reported ranges of <10 mIU/liter until recently. Now, with improved sensitivity, several commercial assays have ranges of <4–5 mIU/liter (Durham, 1985).

Reagent kit manufacturers are required to establish normal, or abnormal, ranges prior to approval by the Food and Drug Administration. Still, manufacturers include the disclaimer that normal ranges should be established in the user's laboratory. It is a difficult task and is rarely done completely in most laboratories. Minimally, laboratories should compare their ranges, even though based on limited data, with the manufacturer's to rule out major systematic bias.

Several practical questions are frequently asked: "How many samples are required?" "How do I calculate the normal range?" "How reliable is the estimate?"

1. Selecting the Normal Population

Without discussion of what is a "normal" person and whether normal is healthy, it is clear that careful selection of a control or reference population against which sick people will be compared is essential and will enhance statistical reliability and clinical utility. Sometimes more than one control group is necessary, depending on the nature of the test. The reference population should be as close in biochemical characteristics as possible to the people for whom the test will be used:

a. Age and sex. Examples include gonadal hormones, which vary with both age and sex and, in addition, may cycle with time. Acid phosphatase used to detect prostate cancer primarily in middle-aged or older men should not necessarily be related to ranges established on 25-year-old house officers.

b. Physiological condition. An extreme example is in the evaluation of α-fetoprotein (AFP) in pregnancy. Since AFP varies with each week of gestation and the test is used between 14 and 21 weeks, this is the equivalent of eight normal range studies! In addition, the range is wide not only because of individual variation but also because the exact date is subject to error. As the sample matrix changes, i.e., from amniotic fluid to serum, another set of ranges is required.

c. Biochemical. Tests that are affected by diet or diurnal variation must also be controlled for the normal range determination.

d. Therapeutic drug use. Subjects should be screened for the presence of therapeutic drugs, including aspirin and birth control pills.

e. Health. Subjects should be at least apparently clinically healthy.

Many hospital and small laboratories rely on the captive audience, laboratory personnel and incoming house officers, for samples. Larger numbers of employees may be available by using samples submitted for routine infection control or health screens. We have obtained specimens for normal range studies by supplying a questionnaire for voluntary information including age, sex, medications, and major or chronic illness. Another group which has been used includes hospital patients with illnesses unrelated to the test being studied, possibly those having a normal biochemical profile. Also, for example, a TSH normal range population might include outpatient samples having normal T_4 and resin uptake values. These populations are flawed by not having clinically verified normality.

2. Calculations

Since the approaches to calculation are statistical in nature, we use a sample population to estimate the range end points of a much larger population. We also expect that the values of the analyte in the population do in fact reflect some (single) central tendency. Without these assumptions the problem is easy; the normal range is simply the range of observations.

A common, but infrequently met, assumption in clinical chemistry is that the frequency distribution of test values is Gaussian (unfortunately, the statistical term ''normal'' for this distribution can cause confusion with the clinical concept of normal) or log Gaussian (i.e., the logarithm of the value follows a Gaussian distribution.) If this assumption is true, then the population can be described by the mean and standard deviation and certain statistical inferences can be made about where a value may lie. A generally accepted normal range has been the 95% confidence limits nominally defined as the mean ± 2 SD.

Authors in clinical literature frequently recommend the use of several nonparametric methods to estimate tolerance intervals or percentiles of a population. Nonparametric estimates do not depend on an *a priori* assumption of the frequency distribution of the population. However, when using nonparametric methods, more observations are necessary to estimate the limits for a given proportion of the population with a given probability. The advantage of these approaches is that even if the underlying distribution is Gaussian, the methods are efficient in establishing the limits. The effect of the assumption and the statistical method on the estimated normal range is well described by Reed *et al.* (1971) with references to standard statistical texts and tables. A few definitions with examples of these approaches should give the reader some idea of how to proceed.

a. Parametric Methods. If the distribution of values is Gaussian, or normal, the mean and SD of observed values estimate the true mean and variance.

The tolerance interval (TI) defines the upper and lower limits which include a specified proportion of the population (e.g., 95%) with a stated probability (e.g., $\gamma = 0.90$). The width of TI depends on the required confidence in the result. For example, it is easier to define a TI if only 50% probability is required. The estimated upper and lower limits of TI come closer to the true upper and lower limits as the number of observations (n) increases. It is also to be noted that this method does not guarantee which 95% of the population is included.

The hypothesis that the distribution is Gaussian can be tested by applying the chi-square test or the Kolmogorov–Smirnov tests, described in standard textbooks. If there are enough observations, simple inspection of a histogram of the distribution may rule out the hypothesis.

A graphic method for assessing whether the Gaussian assumption is true is to plot the cumulative frequency in percent against test value on probability paper. Data are arranged in numerical order from low to high, and the percentage less than and including each value is plotted. A linear graph is consistent with a Gaussian distribution, but often mild curvature is observed. The method is somewhat insensitive to variations in the distribution (Reed *et al.*, 1971).

b. Nonparametric Methods. Nonparametric methods are advised since they require no assumptions about the distribution of data.

Percentile estimates are simple methods for truncating the upper and lower ends of ranked data to include the desired (middle) proportion of the population. For example, if we wished to include 95% of the test population to estimate the normal range, we would simply select as the lower limit the sample value closest to l, where $l = 0.025(n + 1)$. As the upper limit we select the lth highest sample. Our confidence that these limits represent the true limits depends on the number of observations. Tables are available (see Reed *et al.*, 1971) to determine the upper and lower limits for a given confidence. To estimate the 2.5 and 97.5 percentiles with 90% confidence at least 120 samples are required. If this estimate with 70% confidence is adequate, at least 75 samples are required.

Since normal range limits by nonparametric methods rely heavily on the extreme values of the measured population, it is possible that the normal range estimate will be affected by outliers. Investigators have suggested various formulas for disregarding outliers. With very small sample sizes it is often impossible to tell whether an extreme value should be included or whether it represents an individual with undiscovered disease. If possible, the specimen should be repeated to eliminate the possibility of measurement error. Dixon (1953) suggested rejecting a sample as an outlier if the difference between it and the next largest value is greater than one-third of the normal range. If a value is discarded, the range is recalculated. The best way to avoid outliers is to define and select the control population carefully and to include adequate numbers of samples.

In spite of the existence of simplified methods to estimate normal range, the fact remains that it is expensive, sometimes intellectually difficult, and often practically impossible to do thoroughly in a small laboratory. What remains to be done? Many laboratories rely on manufacturers' data and literature values to obtain a reference range. At the very least the laboratory should run as many as possible to check whether values obtained in-house are consistent with the published ranges. Ask the manufacturer for complete information on how their study was done—how many subjects, what kind, and how many laboratories. Often a single laboratory with samples from a limited geographic area will show narrower ranges than the manufacturer's, which includes the effect of different locations as well as any interlaboratory bias. If a laboratory compares a range based on a small number of samples with a published range, there is no valid statistical way to prove with any certainty that the values came from the same population. Individual judgment and consultation with experts may be the only alternatives.

Correlations of new test values with old or with a reference method are often a help in evaluating the normal range.

XII. PROTOCOL DEVELOPMENT: SUMMARY

This chapter has described in some detail how to perform some tests of immunoassay performance. A thorough understanding of the theory and limitations of these experiments aids in the interpretation of test results. It remains to combine the various experiments in an efficient plan to evaluate a new method or to compare methods (Fig. 18). Certain tests may be omitted, depending on the objectives established and on the assay format. The laboratorian may have to redesign a specific test based on the principles presented to adapt to a particular format.

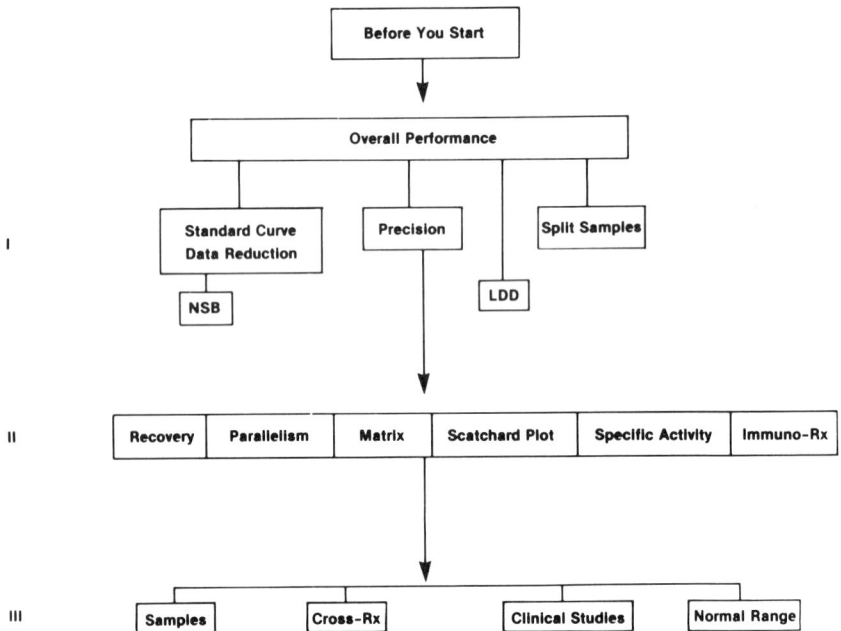

Figure 18. Plan for method evaluation.

Level I: Get acquainted with the assay and solve any technical problems. Inspect standard curves for shape, sensitivity, and NSB. Run replicates of zero to calculate the LDD. Run some patient samples and controls at different levels to compare with assayed values.

Level II: These tests are the heart of the evaluation and will take at least two runs. Run dilutions with blanks on high samples to test parallelism. Recovery and self-displacement studies. Plot a Scatchard plot. Check immunoreactivity.

Level III. On the method tentatively selected, continue to run clinical samples and collect precision data. Establish the normal range.

The first two levels can be accomplished with approximately 300 tubes, barring experimental problems. Many manufacturers will supply the required reagents without charge for a serious evaluator.

The effort in time and reagents for a complete evaluation is extensive. Most laboratories will not undertake such an evaluation unless specific objectives can be established. When the need exists, however, the effort is worth it. When the protocol is followed in ordered stages, data can be accumulated which will support the choice of method and provide the basis for an ongoing quality control program. Even relatively esoteric tests such as cross-reactivity, recovery, and parallelism can be repeated at a later date as needed for problem solving.

REFERENCES

Bernutz, C., Kewenig, M., Horn, K., and Pickardt, C. R. (1985). Detection of thyroid disorders by use of basal thyrotropin values determined with an optimized "sandwich" enzyme immunoassay. *Clin. Chem.* **31**, 289–292.

Bremner, W. S., and Chase, G. D. (1980). Some concepts of RIA theory, data reduction, and quality control. IV. Binding mechanism and nonlinear Scatchard plots. *Ligand Quarterly* **3**, 21–27.

Chervu, L. R., and Murty, D. R. K. (1975). Radiolabeling of antigens: procedures and assessment of properties. *Semin. Nucl. Med.* **5**, 157–172.

Dixon, W. J. (1953). Processing data for outliers. *Biometrics* **9**, 74.

Dotti, C., and Castagnetti, C. (1978). Non-specific count subtraction in radioimmunoassay (a criticism). *Ric. Clin. Lab.* **8**, 301–311.

Durham, A. P. (1985). The upper limit of normal for thyrotropin is 3 or 4 milli-int. units/L. *Clin. Chem.* **31**, 296–298.

Edelman, G. M. (1973). Antibody structure and molecular immunology. *Science* **180**, 830–840.

Ehrlich, P. H., and Moyle, W. R. (1984). Specificity considerations in cooperative immunoassays. *Clin. Chem.* **30**, 1523–1532.

Ekins, R. (1981). The "precision profile": its use in RIA assessment and design. *Ligand Quarterly* **4**, 33–44.

Englebienne, P., and Slegein, G. (1983). Estimation of the specific activity of radioiodinated gonadotrophins: comparison of three methods. *J. Immunol. Methods* **56**, 135–140.

Feldkamp, C. S., Chapin, E., and Shearer, G. (1977). Blanking in insulin radioimmunoassay. *Clin. Chem.* **23**, 1167 (abstr.)

Feldman, H., Rodbard, D., and Levine, D. (1972). Mathematical theory of cross-reactive radioim-munoassay and ligand-binding systems at equilibrium. *Anal. Biochem.* **45,** 530–556.

Fernandez, A. A., Stevenson, G. W., Abraham, G. E., and Chiamori, N.Y. (1983). Interrelations of the various mathematical approaches to radioimmunoassay. *Clin. Chem.* **29,** 284–289.

Galen, R. S., and Gambino, S. R. (1975). "Beyond Normality. The Predictive Value and Efficiency of Medical Diagnoses." John Wiley & Sons, New York.

Garrett, P. E. (1985). Method evaluation I: screening assays with package insert data. *J. Clin. Immunoassay* **8,** 57–62.

Garrett, P. E., and Krouwer, J. S. (1985). Method evaluation II: precision and sensitivity considera-tions. *J. Clin. Immunoassay* **8,** 165–168.

Gendrel, D., Feinstein, M. D., and Grenier, J. (1981). Falsely elevated serum thyrotropin (TSH) in newborn infants: transfer from mothers to infants of a factor interfering in the TSH radioim-munoassay. *J. Clin. Endocrinol. Metab.* **52,** 62–65.

Goldstein, J., and Vanhaelst, L. (1973). Influence of thyrotropin-free serum on the radioim-munoassay of human thyrotropin. *Clin. Chim. Acta* **49,** 141–146.

Henry, R. J., Cannon, D. C., and Winkleman, J. W. (1974). "Clinical Chemistry." Harper & Row, New York.

Hoffman, K. L. (1985). Optimization of sandwich immunometric assay. *J. Clin. Immunoassay* **8,** 237–244.

Hollemans, H. J. G., and Bertina, R. M. (1975). Scatchard plot and heterogeneity in binding affinity of labeled and unlabeled ligand. *Clin. Chem.* **21,** 1769–1773.

Homsher, R. (1985). Effect of data reduction on accuracy assessment in an enzyme immunoassay. *J. Clin. Immunoassay* **8,** 230–233.

Perlstein, M. T. (1979). Parallelism: effects of protein matrixes and mathematical treatment of data. *Ligand Quarterly* **2,** 6–8.

Perlstein, M. T., Chan, D. W., and Bill, M. J. (1980). Parallelism: a useful tool for troubleshooting. *Ligand Quarterly* **3,** 34–36.

Reed, A. H., Henry, R. J., and Mason, W. B. (1971). Influence of statistical method used on the resulting estimate of normal range. *Clin. Chem.* **17,** 275–284.

Rodbard, D., Rayford, P. L., Cooper, J. A., and Ross, G. T. (1968). Statistical quality control of radioimmunoassays. *J. Clin. Endocrinol.* **28,** 1412–1218.

Rodbard, D., Ruder, H. J., Vaitukaitis, J., and Jacobs, H. S. (1971). Mathematical analysis of kinetics of radioligand assays: improved sensitivity obtained by delayed addition of labeled ligand. *J. Clin. Endocrinol.* **33,** 343–355.

Scatchard, G. (1949). The attraction of proteins for small molecules and ions. *Ann. N.Y. Acad. Sci.* **51,** 660–672.

Seidman, J. G., Leder, A., Nau, M., Norman, B., and Leder, P. (1978). Antibody diversity. *Science* **202,** 11–17

Seth, J., Kellett, H. A., Caldwell, G., Sweeting, V. M., Beckett, G. J., Gow, S. M., and Toft, A. D. (1984). A sensitive immunoradiometric assay for serum thyroid stimulating hormone: a replacement for the thyrotrophin releasing hormone test? *Br. Med. J.* **289,** 1334–1336.

Smith, S. W. (1985). Application of the Scatchard plot to radioimmunoassay I: theoretical considera-tions. *J. Clin. Immunoassay* **8,** 52–55.

Smith, S. W., and Feldkamp, C. S. (1979). Qualitative features of Scatchard plots: positive cur-vature. *Ligand Quarterly* **2**(4), 37–40.

Stockigt, V. R., Stevens, V., White, E. L., and Barlow, J. W. (1983). "Unbound analog" radioim-munoassays for free thyroxin measure the albumin-bound hormone fraction. *Clin. Chem.* **27,** 1408–1410.

Tonegawa, S., Steinberg, C., Dube, S., and Bernardini, A. (1974). Evidence for somatic generation of antibody diversity. *Proc. Natl. Acad. Sci. U.S.A.* **71,** 4027–4031.

Vladutiu, A. O., Sulewski, J. M., Pudlak, K. A., and Stull, C. G. (1982). Heterophilic antibodies interfering with radioimmunoassay. A false-positive pregnancy test. *JAMA J. Am. Med. Assoc.* **248,** 2489–2490.

Walker, W. H. C., and Kean, P. M. (1977). Theoretical aspects of radioimmunoassay. *In* "Handbook of Radioimmunoassay" (G. E. Abraham, ed.), Vol. V, pp. 87–130. Dekker, New York.

Yallow, R. S. (1980). Radioimmunoassay. *Annu. Rev. Biophys. Bioeng.* **9,** 327–345.

Zettner, A. (1973). Principles of competitive binding assays (saturation analysis). I. Equilibrium techniques. *Clin. Chem.* **19,** 699–705.

Chapter 4

Clinical Validation of Immunoassays:
A Well-Designed Approach
to a Clinical Study

Mark H. Zweig

E. Arthur Robertson

Clinical Chemistry Service
Clinical Pathology Department
Clinical Center
National Institutes of Health
Bethesda, Maryland 20892

Pathology Associates of Southwestern
Michigan, P.C.
Benton Harbor, Michigan 49022

I. INTRODUCTION

Why write about establishing the clinical value of a test? We write about it because commonsense principles are quite often ignored or overlooked in assessing the clinical usefulness of a test (Beck, 1982; Kassirer and Pauker, 1978; Ransohoff and Feinstein, 1978; Zweig and Robertson, 1982). Furthermore, although concepts such as predictive value and efficiency are helpful, they are frequently misunderstood and used inappropriately. Such errors lead to over- or underestimates of a test's usefulness, misleading comparisons of tests, and inappropriate conclusions about the clinical application of individual tests.

This chapter will discuss how to determine a test's clinical value and how to optimize its usefulness. This process is most readily implemented with new tests having a few specific applications, but these principles can also be applied to existing tests where specific clinical goals are defined, either to compare tests to each other, to optimize their use individually, or to determine whether the information they provide is redundant. Failure to consider carefully what the clinical question being addressed is and to evaluate properly the test's performance in the relevant setting can lead to improper use of the test. This may result in testing the wrong patient population, duplicating information, replacing a superior test with an inferior one, or using the wrong decision level to distinguish between affected and unaffected individuals. The consequences range from wasted resources at best through harm to people at worst. In the following discussion we will first deal with overall design of a study to evaluate a test, with attention to defining the clinical question. Then we will cover selection of appropriate subjects to study, the role and importance of the "gold standard" to classify the subjects accurately, how to test all subjects properly, examination of test performance and comparison of tests to one another, choice of the optimal conditions for clinical application, and the relationship to existing tests.

II. ELEMENTS OF A WELL-DESIGNED STUDY

A. Defining the Clinical Question

The medical usefulness of a test depends, in the final analysis, on its success in answering a question of clinical consequence—in providing information which makes a difference in the way a patient is managed. Simply providing information which is redundant, merely unusual, or irrelevant to medical management does not make a test clinically useful. Accordingly, the evaluation of a test's medical usefulness must focus on its success in answering a specific question of consequence in a particular clinical setting.

Generally the clinical question will refer to a group of apparently similar patients grouped together on the basis of the information available before the test under evaluation is performed. The clinical question which the test is expected to answer will ask to which management subgroup individual patients belong. For example, a radioimmunoassay for apolipoprotein A-I might be used to answer the question, "Of male patients referred for diagnostic coronary angiograms for chest pain, which ones will have greater than 50% stenosis of at least one vessel? (Maciejko *et al.,* 1983). In this case the original group of apparently similar patients consists of males with "chest pain or suspected coronary artery disease" judged significant enough by their physicians to warrant coronary angiography. The test is asked to divide the patients into two management subgroups: those who do not have greater than 50% stenosis of any vessel (and thus would not be subjected to angiography at all if their freedom from stenosis could be predicted ahead of time) and those who have greater than 50% stenosis of at least one vessel (and thus would be given either medical or surgical therapy, depending on the nature of their angiographic findings).

A radioimmunoassay for serum angiotensin-converting enzyme activity might be expected to answer the question, "Among patients with hypercalcemia, which ones have sarcoidosis?" The group of apparently similar patients share the common characteristic of hypercalcemia. The test under evaluation attempts to divide them into subgroups which would receive different treatments—those with sarcoidosis and those with some other cause of hypercalcemia (such as malignancy or hyperparathyroidism) (Lufkin *et al.*, 1983).

B. Selecting a Study Sample from the Population of Interest

When adequately formulated, the clinical question defines the population relevant to the test evaluation. From this clinical population, a sample of individuals must be chosen for the study. These individuals must be representative of the larger population of clinical interest, since the goal of the study is to reach conclusions which can be extrapolated to this larger population.

Ideally, subjects should be chosen by a random process to prevent biases in subject selection which could compromise the validity of the study's conclusions. Selection procedures based on convenience are likely to produce nonrepresentative samples. Using only those patients admitted early on weekdays might select for electively admitted patients to the exclusion of emergency admissions. Using only patients for whom the laboratory had a large amount of leftover serum would tend to exclude small and pediatric patients. Whenever nonrandom selection procedures are used, a nonrepresentative sample may be obtained. The nature and magnitude of the biases which may result should be carefully considered.

The test result or the testing procedure must not be allowed to influence the selection of subjects. Excluding patients with unexpected, equivocal, or discordant results is likely to make the test appear more useful than it actually is, since the problem cases are left out. A retrospective study using only patients who actually had their test results reported excludes patients who could not be successfully tested for various reasons, again possibly inflating the apparent usefulness of the test.

Choosing subjects prospectively before testing begins guards against the biases introduced when the test result directly or indirectly influences the selection of subjects. One selection technique which avoids many biases is to include a consecutive series of all patients meeting the definition of the clinical group of interest until a predetermined number of subjects have been obtained. Once chosen, subjects should not be dropped from the study. If some patients do not complete the study (because of technical errors, analytical interferences, death, loss to follow-up, etc.), they must be accounted for in the final analysis of the data. The uncertainty and possible biases which the lost subjects cause in the study's conclusions must be analyzed and reported.

C. Determining the True Answer to the Clinical Question

For each subject, the study must obtain two basic pieces of information: the result of the test under evaluation and the true answer to the clinical question. How to determine these pieces of information in an accurate, unbiased manner will be discussed in this and the next sections.

The validity of the test evaluation is limited by the accuracy with which the true answer to the clinical question is determined. Consider the hypothetical situation in Fig. 1. The clinical question is, "Has this patient presenting at the emergency room with an acute psychiatric disorder used marijuana recently?" The routine test is sensitive enough to detect only 70% of the recent drug users; 30% of the marijuana users have falsely negative results. The routine test also suffers from various interferences, leading to false positive results in 30% of nonusers. Test I represents a new test which is being evaluated. In actuality it manifests excellent sensitivity and specificity, giving positive results in all recent marijuana users and negative results in all nonusers. If, however, instead of independently and accurately determining the drug-use status of each patient, the patients are simply classed as users or nonusers on the basis of the routine test's results, test I will appear to perform poorly, misclassifying 30% of the patients. In this case a perfect test appears to perform poorly simply because the clinical question was not answered accurately for each patient; that is, the gold standard used for comparison was inadequate.

The opposite bias can also result from use of inadequate gold standards. Test II in Fig. 1 performs even more poorly than the routine test, yielding false negative results in 40% of the marijuana users and false positive results in 40% of the nonusers. If, however, the routine test's results are accepted as correct and test II

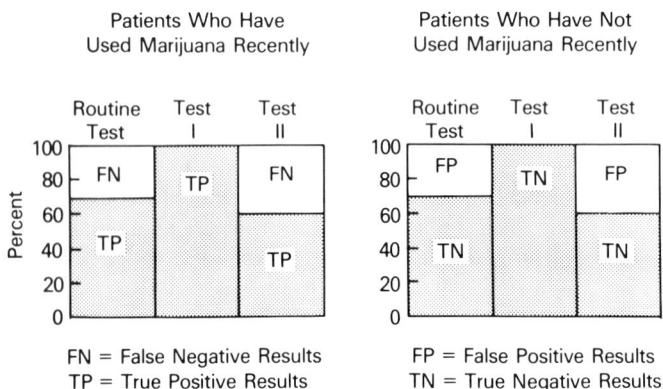

Figure 1. Hypothetical performance of three tests for marijuana use in two subgroups of patients, one of which has used marijuana recently and one which has not. It is assumed that the routine test gives correct results in 70% of subjects.

is judged on this basis, test II will appear to misclassify only 10% of the patients—and will have a better apparent performance than test I!

This can occur in several ways in clinical practice. In evaluating a test for acute myocardial infarction, if the patients are classifed on the basis of EKG data alone or even a combination of history, EKG findings, and some cardiac enzyme results (a "routine workup"), the diagnosis may still be inaccurate and thus distort the apparent performance of the new test. In the case of a cancer tumor marker, if the gold standard (diagnosis or staging, etc.) is based on clinical findings rather than surgical and/or tissue data, then the gold standard may be inaccurate and bias the apparent value of the marker. If an amniotic fluid marker for fetal lung maturity is compared to an existing imperfect marker, then even if the new marker is perfect, it will appear imperfect. The gold standard against which the new marker should be compared is the actual presence or absence of respiratory distress syndrome in newborns delivered within a short time of measurement of the marker.

Because the validity of a clinical evaluation's conclusions is critically dependent on accurate determination of the answer to the clinical question for each subject, routine clinical diagnoses are likely to be inadequate for test evaluation studies. Definitive determination of a patient's true clinical subgroup may require such procedures as biopsy, surgical exploration, autopsy examination, angiography, or long-term follow-up of response to therapy and clinical outcome. Such rigorous patient workups may well add considerable cost to the test evaluation. However, an "inexpensive" clinical evaluation may prove very costly in the long run if its erroneous conclusions lead to improper test utilization or improper patient management.

In many situations of clinical interest, it is difficult to obtain an independent accurate diagnosis of the patient's true clinical condition. This problem can sometimes be resolved by a longer-term clinical follow-up of the subjects to determine which ones respond favorably to the treatment of interest. Even when the correct diagnosis can easily be established, a study correlating test results with the clinical course may provide a more useful clinical evaluation than one which merely correlates test results with patient diagnoses. Although diagnostic categories often predict complications and therapeutic responses, the most relevant assessment of a test is in terms of its ability to determine optimal patient management. Thus the lack of a definitive diagnosis does not necessarily prevent a valid assessment of a test's clinical utility.

To avoid bias in evaluating a test's clinical performance, the answer to the clinical question must also be determined independently of the test under investigation or any existing tests being examined or used for comparison. Bias can be introduced by including either a test being evaluated or a closely related test in the diagnostic criteria. Obviously, the new test(s) itself should not be included in the criteria used to classify the subjects. This source of bias, however, can occur for existing tests in a subtle way and escape notice. If a test for the MB iso-enzyme of creative kinase (CK-MB) is being evaluated for the diagnosis of myocardial infarction, it may seem logical to compare its performance to the performance of existing tests such as lactate dehydrogenase isoenzyme 1 (LD-1), total LD, aminotransferase activity, or some combination of "cardiac en-zymes." Even though the existing tests are not being evaluated primarily as new markers *per se,* their apparent performance "revealed" by the evaluation is biased by their inclusion in the diagnostic criteria. If their performance is biased, then any comparison between them and new test(s) will be biased. These existing tests, then, must not be included in the diagnostic criteria if their performance is to be evaluated and compared to that of new tests.

Suppose we were evaluating the performance of a test for glycosylated hemo-globin in terms of its ability to reflect overall blood glucose control over a period of months in subjects with diabetes. We might evaluate the test by judging the level of glucose control which the patients had on the basis of frequent measure-ments of blood glucose, urine glucose, urine ketones, and clinical data. Howev-er, it would not be appropriate to pull out average blood glucose concentration and compare its performance to glycosylated hemoglobin since the classification of subjects was strongly influenced by those concentrations.

Tests closely related to the test(s) being evaluated should also be excluded from the diagnostic criteria. Thus, in an evaluation of the effectiveness of an immunochemical assay for LD-1 in the diagnosis of acute myocardial infarction, the related tests for hydroxybutyrate dehydrogenase or heat-stable LD could not be used to establish the diagnosis, since they both are approximate measures of LD-1 activity.

To help ensure that the answer to the clinical question is not influenced by the result of the test under evaluation, it is preferable to answer the clinical question blindly, that is, without knowledge of the test result. Furthermore, the criteria for answering the clinical question (that is, for classifying each patient into one or the other of the management subgroups) should be as objective as feasible. When the classification must rest on subjective evaluation of clinical or morphological patterns such as radionuclide scans or bone marrow smears, it is desirable that the decision for each patient reflect the consensus of multiple experts who each interpret the material blindly and independently.

D. Testing the Study Subjects

To avoid possible biases, the test under evaluation should be performed blind-ly, that is, without knowledge of the subject's clinical status, on the part of the person carrying out the test. Ideally, the testing should be done prospectively before the clinical question has been answered. When the person doing the testing is aware of the answer to the clinical question, the door is opened for subtle biases. Results that do not fit the clinical status might be selectively repeated or perhaps rejected on the basis of supposed technical difficulties or interfering factors.

When multiple tests are being compared in the same study, all tests should be performed on all subjects. Furthermore, each subject should have all the tests done at the same point in the course of his or her illness. No two sets of subjects are identical. Even unbiased truly random samples differ from sample to sample because of statistical variations. In addition, many actual samples suffer from unrecognized bias in the selection process. Thus, if tests being evaluated are not applied to the same group of subjects, observed differences in test performance may reflect differences in the subjects tested rather than differences in actual test efficacy. Similarly, if two tests are applied to the same patient at different points in the course of the patient's illness, the apparent superiority of one test over the other may simply indicate that the disease had reached a more "diagnosable" stage when the later testing was done.

Practical evaluation of a test's clinical usefulness requires consideration of the time, equipment, and skill required to perform it. A test which requires hours to perform will provide little help with an urgent therapeutic decision which must be made within minutes. Even if the clinical answers it provides are accurate, a test may find little clinical acceptance if its cost or complexity is out of proportion to the importance of the information it provides.

Conducting the testing in real time in a production clinical laboratory provides an opportunity for the study to evaluate the practicality as well as the clinical efficacy of the test. On the other hand, a test developer may wish to evaluate the clinical effectiveness of a complex, time-consuming, or expensive test in a research setting to determine whether or not to invest in efforts to make the procedure simpler, quicker, and less expensive.

E. Evaluating Test Performance

Performance is commonly assessed by examining the ability of the test to correctly classify individuals into two subgroups, for example, a subgroup of individuals affected by some disease (and thus needing treatment) and a second subgroup of unaffected individuals. If there is no overlap in test results from these two subgroups, then the test can identify all individuals correctly, that is, distinguish the two subgroups perfectly. However, if there is some overlap in the test results for the two subgroups, then the test cannot distinguish them perfectly. This raises the question, How much deviation is there from perfection?

1. Sensitivity and Specificity

Let us define the ability to identify affected individuals as sensitivity and the ability to recognize unaffected individuals as specificity and express these abilities as percentages or decimal fractions. A perfect test would exhibit both a sensitivity and a specificity of 100% or 1.0. Tests are rarely perfect. It would be rather unusual for a test to exhibit a sensitivity and a specificity of 100% at the same time. Often, we hear or read that a particular test has a particular sensitivity and specificity. In reality, there is not just one sensitivity or specificity for a test, but rather a continuum of sensitivities and specificities. By varying the decision level (or "decision point," "upper limit of normal," "cutoff value," "reference value," etc.) any sensitivity from 0 to 100% can be obtained. Each of these sensitivities will have a corresponding specificity. Sensitivity and specificity occur, then, in pairs. The test's performance is reflected in the pairs that can occur; not all pairs are possible for a particular test. A given test will have one set of sensitivity–specificity pairs in one clinical situation, but may have a different set of pairs when applied to another clinical situation where the group tested is different.

The spectrum of pairs exhibited by a test in a given clinical setting characterizes or describes the performance of the test. Often test users implicitly assume that one sensitivity–specificity pair characterizes a test because they accept a conventional, often arbitrarily chosen, upper limit of normal as the single correct decision level for that test for all circumstances. They implicitly accept the corresponding sensitivity–specificity pair as the correct one for the test. This, however, is actually only one of multiple possible operating points for the test. When the concept of varying the decision level (operating point) to generate a spectrum of sensitivity–specificity pairs is understood, the issues become: How good are the pairs? Which pairs work best for the circumstances in which the test is to be used?

2. Receiver Operating Characteristic (ROC) Curves

To answer these questions, we first need a way to represent and deal with all these different possible operating points and their resultant performance characteristics. The ROC curve graphically displays the entire spectrum of a given test's performance for a particular sample group of affected and unaffected subjects. Figure 2 contains a hypothetical frequency distribution histogram at the top and the corresponding ROC curve below. The ROC curve plots the true positive (TP) rate or percentage as a function of the false positive (FP) rate or percentage as the decision level is varied. The true positive rate is the same as sensitivity and is equal to the number of *affected* individuals with a "positive" result divided by the total number of affected individuals. The true positive rate is also equal to $1 -$ false negative (FN) rate. The false positive rate is the fraction of *unaffected* individuals who nevertheless have a "positive" test result and is therefore related to specificity, or the ability of the test to correctly identify unaffected individuals [specificity = true negative (TN) rate = number of unaffected individuals with "negative" results/total number of unaffected individuals = $1 -$ false positive rate].

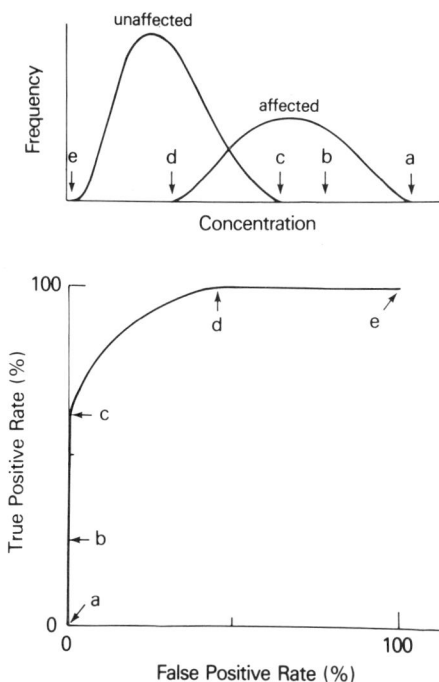

Figure 2. (Top) Hypothetical frequency distribution curve. (Bottom) Receiver operating characteristic curve corresponding to data in top panel, generated by varying the decision level and then plotting the resulting pairs of true and false positive rates. Arrows at a to e mark points corresponding to decision levels in top panel. The curve from c to d describes the test's performance in the crucial overlap region.

Both the TP and FP rates depend on the decision level chosen. Both rates also depend on the clinical setting, as reflected by the study population chosen. The FP rate is influenced by the type of nondiseased subjects included in the study group. If, for example, the nondiseased subjects are all healthy blood donors who are free of any signs or symptoms, the test may appear to have a much lower FP rate than if the nondiseased subjects are persons who clinically resemble those who actually have the disease. Like the FP rate, the TP rate also depends on the study group. A test used to detect cancer may have a higher TP rate when applied to patients who have active or advanced disease than when applied to patients who have stable or limited disease. This dependence of TP and FP rates on the study population is the reason why an ROC curve must be generated for each clinical situation.

Each point on the ROC curve represents a pair of true and false positive rates corresponding to some decision level. In Fig. 2, the left-hand curve of the frequency histogram (top) represents results from unaffected individuals and the right-hand curve is derived from affected individuals. The ROC curve is derived from the data in the frequency histogram, so the first step is to obtain the test results from both the affected group and the unaffected group. True positive rates are calculated using the results from the affected individuals, while false positive rates are generated from the unaffected individuals' data. The ROC curve is constructed by varying the decision level from the highest test result down to zero, resulting in true and false positive rates which vary continuously. The decision level at point a in Fig. 2 is higher than any observed results (see top), so at that decision level, none of the results is "positive" and both true and false positive rates are zero (see bottom). As the decision level is lowered from a to b, some of the affected individuals have positive results but none of the unaffected individuals does, so the true positive rate rises while the false positive rate remains zero. Point c shows the highest true positive rate achievable (with these data) with the false positive rate still at zero. This is the edge of the overlap region (c to d). At c the ROC curve leaves the Y axis because if the decision level is lowered further, some unaffected individuals will have falsely positive results. At decision level d all affected individuals have positive test results, so the true positive rate reaches 100%, at the expense of some percentage of false positives. This is the other edge of the crucial overlap region. The portion of the curve from c to d (where it has left the Y axis but not yet intercepted the true positive = 100% horizontal line) describes the overlap region. From decision level d to e, false positive rates increase as more and more results from unaffected individuals are incorrectly classified as positive.

The complete ROC curve summarizes the clinical performance of the test by displaying the paired true and false positive rates for all possible decision levels. Good clinical performance of a test is characterized by a high true positive rate and a low false positive rate. Accordingly, as test performance improves, the ROC curve will move upward (toward higher true positive rates) and to the left (toward lower false positive rates). A perfect test would achieve a 100% true positive rate with no false positives. Thus, its ROC curve would rise vertically to the (0, 100) point in the upper left corner and then move horizontally to the right along the horizontal line representing true positive rate = 100% to the (100, 100) point in the upper right corner. Conversely, for a clinically useless test, which gives similar results for subjects with and without the condition, the true and false positive rates would be identical for any given decision level. Therefore, the ROC curve would be a diagonal between the lower left and upper right corners, representing the line where the true positive rate always equals the false positive rate.

The ROC curve can also be constructed as a plot of true positive rate (sensitivity) versus true negative rate (specificity) instead of false positive rate (1−specificity). This produces a mirror image of the curve shown in Fig. 2, flipping the curve to the right side with the perfect point being the upper right corner instead of the upper left corner.

The ROC curve, then, provides a comprehensive picture of the test's performance capabilities at all possible operating points (decision levels). It does this without the need to choose a decision level or establish a normal range in advance. Furthermore, it allows complete comparisons of any number of tests to one another over all possible decision levels.

3. Comparing Tests

Besides being valuable in evaluating a single test by demonstrating the complete spectrum of its intrinsic performance, the ROC curve is extremely useful in comparing tests to one another. Even if we are evaluating only a single new test, comparisons to existing tests are often inherent in the evaluation process. ROC curves provide an elegantly simple means of demonstrating the relative performance of multiple tests.

To get a valid comparison of the performance of different tests, all tests should be examined under the same conditions. This means that, as mentioned above, the diseased and nondiseased patients should be the same for all tests, and individual subjects should all be tested at the same point in their clinical course. Furthermore, either the TP rates or the FP rates must be the same for all tests. If, for example, test A has TP and FP rates of 98 and 30%, respectively, and test B has rates of 70 and 2%, it is difficult to judge which is performing better. Test A is more sensitive (TP rate of 98 versus 70%), but test B is more specific (FP rate of 2 versus 30%). From these data it cannot be determined what the FP rate for test B would be if a decision level were chosen so that it, like test A, had a TP rate of 98%. If decision levels for each test were chosen to achieve equal TP rates for the two tests, they could then be compared directly on the basis of the corresponding FP rates. (The TP rate chosen should generally not be 100%, since the decision level that would just achieve a 100% TP rate usually cannot be determined accurately with samples of practical size.)

A second and more comprehensive way of comparing tests is to compare them at every TP rate by plotting the ROC curves for all the tests on the same graph. If the ROC curve for one test is uniformly above and to the left of the ROC curve for a second test, the first test will have a lower FP rate than the second test for any chosen TP rate.

The ROC curves of Fig. 3 illustrate the ambiguity involved in comparing tests when neither the TP nor the FP rates are equal. Consider the above case in which test A has a TP rate of 98% and an FP rate of 30%, while test B has a TP rate of 70% and an FP rate of 2%. If the clinical performance of the two tests were equivalent, they would share a single ROC curve. This situation is illustrated in Fig. 3, left. Test B could have achieved the same TP and FP rates as test A if a different decision level had been used. In fact, either test could have achieved any of the pairs of TP and FP rates on the common ROC curve simply by

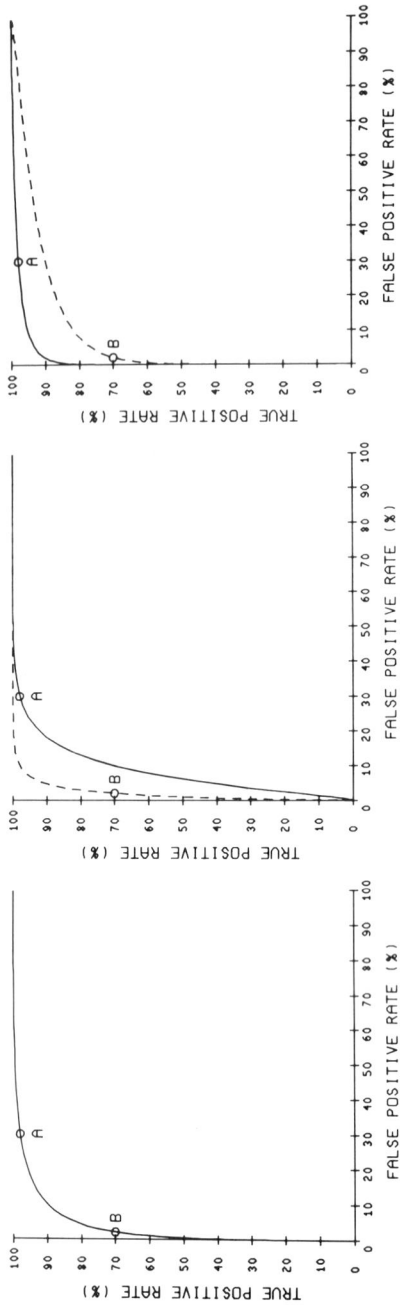

Figure 3. Hypothetical ROC curves showing three possible relations between tests A and B. In each case, test A exhibits a true positive rate of 98% and a false positive rate of 30%, while test B exhibits a true positive rate of 70% and a false positive rate of 2%. (Left) Both tests have identical ROC curves and thus equivalent diagnostic abilities. (Middle) Test B has a better ROC curve. (Right) Test A has a better curve.

changing the decision level. Thus the two tests may in fact share a single ROC curve but initially appear to be different because the two decision levels used place the tests at different points on the curve; that is, the operating conditions were not comparable. On the other hand, the two tests may perform very differently, with test B clearly superior, as illustrated in Fig. 3, center. Regardless of the decision level chosen for test A, it cannot achieve a TP rate of 70% with an FP rate of only 2%, as did test B. In fact, when test A's TP is 70%, its FP rate is 10%. Similarly, the true and false positive rates given originally would be equally consistent with the situation show in Fig. 3, right, where test A is clearly superior. These examples illustrate how the use of ROC curves avoids the ambiguity which may occur when tests are compared using only one decision level for each different test.

There are two ways, then, to compare tests at comparable decision levels. The first, setting a single TP rate and then comparing on the basis of the FP rates (or vice versa), is the simplest but incomplete. Since the comparison is made at only one decision level for each test, one gets only one look at the tests' relative performances. The actual relationship between the tests can vary over the decision level continuum so that, while test A may look similar to test B at one sensitivity–specificity, it may look very different at another. For example, in Fig. 3, center, at an FP rate of 40% both tests exhibit similar sensitivities (nearly 100%). However, at an FP rate of 10%, the two tests have very different sensitivities. The second approach to achieving comparable decision levels, using ROC curves, obviates this problem by comparing the tests at *all* decision levels. Another advantage of ROC curve analysis is that test comparison can be performed without having to choose any specific decision level or "upper limit."

Figure 4 shows the ROC curves for two tests, myoglobin and CK-MB, demonstrating their respective abilities to identify myocardial infarction among persons with chest pain admitted to a coronary care unit. These data are derived from measurements of the two analytes in serum obtained 20 h after the onset of pain. It is obvious by visual inspection that CK-MB has a far superior ROC curve. The CK-MB curve is very close to "perfect," in fact, in that it comes close to going through the ideal point (0, 100) in the upper left-hand corner. Aside from regions where the curves are superimposed (either when both FP rates are essentially zero or when both TP rates approach 100%), CK-MB exhibits a lower FP rate for any given TP rate. Similarly, CK-MB exhibits a higher TP rate for any given FP rate than does myoglobin. Clearly, CK-MB is more effective at classifying subjects with chest pain admitted to a coronary care unit with chest pain and sampled at 20 h after the onset of pain. This judgment can be made with confidence because the entire spectrum of performance possibilities is shown here in terms of all the sensitivity–specificity pairs which each test could achieve in this clinical setting. No selection of an "upper limit of normal" or "reference

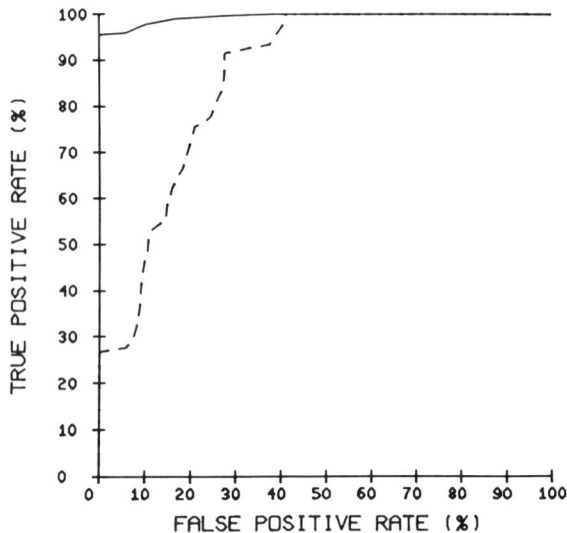

Figure 4. ROC curves for serum myoglobin (dotted line) and CK-MB (solid line) concentrations 20 h after the onset of chest pain in patients suspected of having a myocardial infarction.

range'' was required to appreciate either the performance of CK-MB or its superiority over myoglobin. Neither were any determinations in healthy subjects required.

In the case of myocardial infarction, as with many other conditions, the disease evolves over time. This time factor is critical in identifying persons with infarction among subjects with chest pain and the suspicion of infarction. Figure 4 exhibits the performance data for the two tests when the blood sample was obtained at one particular time interval after the onset of chest pain, 20 h. It happens that the highest serum concentrations of CK-MB in acute myocardial infarction appear in the vicinity of 16–22 h after the onset of chest pain (Van Steirteghem *et al.*, 1982). During this period the difference between subjects with and without actual infarcts is greatest, and so the test is most powerful at distinguishing the two subgroups. On the other hand, myoglobin concentrations in serum are not very different in the two subgroups at this point in the evolution of the disease but are quite different at earlier intervals after the onset of pain. ROC curves of these two tests at 8 h after the onset of pain show that myoglobin is superior to CK-BB (Van Steirteghem *et al.*, 1982). It is useful, in such situations, to plot the ROC curves of a single test *at different times* in the course of the disease on single graph. This reveals the time or times at which the test is most powerful at making the desired classification. Such a plot for myoglobin at 8, 18, and 60 h shows that the ROC curves become progressively inferior as the time interval from onset of pain increases from 8 to 60 h (Fig. 5). By sampling frequently and by measuring myoglobin, total creatine kinase, CK-MB, and CK-BB in each sample, ROC curves for each test were constructed at 24 different intervals up to 96 h after the onset of pain. This revealed the comparative abilities of these four tests at different times, showing, for example, that myoglobin was most effective at 8 h, that all three creatine kinase tests were very effective at 18–20 h, and that total creatine kinase was the most effective test at 48 h (Van Steirteghem *et al.*, 1982). Thus ROC curves can be used to determine the time in the course of a disease when a test performs best, as well as to compare multiple tests to one another at a given time.

Once the study population has been tested and the results plotted as ROC curves, it will be evident by visual inspection which test is best and what sensitivity–specificity pairs each test can achieve. The next step, discussed below, is to select a decision level or operating point to use when actually putting the test into use clinically. This phase involves considering the prevalence of the condition in the population the test will be used for, costs of false results, and parameters such as predictive value which help us understand the significance of test results for individual patients. At this point, let us consider the derivation and role of predictive value and efficiency.

4. Predictive Value and Efficiency

Sensitivity, specificity, predictive value, and efficiency are all commonly used to describe test performance. How are they related to each other? Are they the

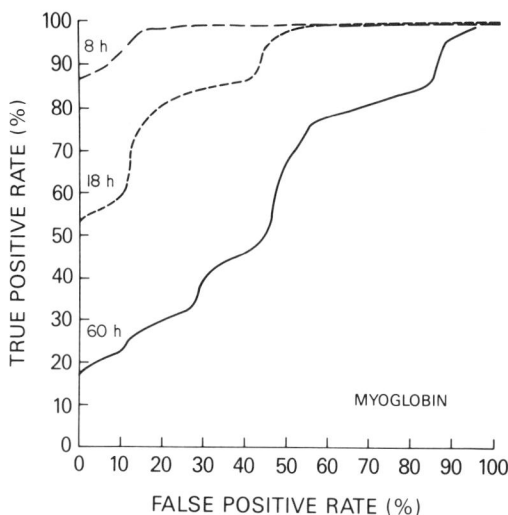

Figure 5. ROC curves for serum myoglobin at 8, 18, and 60 h after the onset of chest pain in patients suspected of having a myocardial infarction.

same or different? If different, which are better? This section will attempt to put these parameters and their roles in perspective.

Sensitivity and specificity vary as the decision level varies, as discussed above. However, neither varies with the prevalence of the condition in the population. (The prevalence of a condition is the fraction of the population which has the condition.) In contrast, predictive value and efficiency vary with both decision level and prevalence. Sensitivity describes how well the test recognizes diseased members of a population; specificity describes how well the test recognizes subjects without the disease. For a particular population, predictive value describes the likely meaning or correctness of positive (or negative) test results. Efficiency tells what percentage of all test results will be correct for a particular population. This is more clearly illustrated by the four-cell matrix in Fig. 6. The four cells contain the four possible kinds of results: true positives, true negatives, false positives, false negatives. Sensitivity (''positivity in disease'') is calculated by dividing the number of true positive results by the total number of affected individuals, using data from the two cells on the *left*. Similarly, specificity (''negativity in health'') is calculated by dividing the number of true negative results by the total number of unaffected individuals, using the data on the *right*-hand two cells. Predictive value of a positive result describes the fraction of positive results which are true positives and thus is calculated by dividing the number of true positives by the total number of positive results, using data from the *upper* two cells. Similarly, the predictive value of a negative result is the fraction of negative results which are from truly unaffected individuals and is calculated from the *lower* two cells.

If the prevalence of the disease or condition in the population shifts, the relative numbers of individuals occurring on the right and left sides of this matrix

		Disease or Condition present	Disease or Condition absent
Test Result	"positive"	TP	FP
	"negative"	FN	TN

$$PV(+) = \frac{TP}{TP + FP} \times 100$$

$$PV(-) = \frac{TN}{FN + TN} \times 100$$

$$\text{Sensitivity} = \frac{TP}{TP + FN} \times 100$$

$$\text{Specificity} = \frac{TN}{FP + TN} \times 100$$

Figure 6. Four-cell matrix showing four possible types of test results and formulas for calculating performance parameters. PV(+), Predictive value of a positive test result; PV(−), predictive value of a negative test result.

```
                            Disease or Condition

                        present              absent


              "positive"      980              19,800
        Test
        Result
              "negative"       20              79,200


        Total subjects = 100,000

        Prevalence = 1%

        Sensitivity = 98%

        Specificity = 80%

        PV(+) =       980         X 100 = 4.7%
                  980 + 19,800
```

Figure 7. Four-cell matrix for hypothetical test with a prevalence of 1%, sensitivity of 98%, and specificity of 80%.

will change. If the spectrum of the disease does not change, shifts from right to left or from left to right do not change the proportions of individuals falling in the upper or lower cells. Thus, sensitivity and specificity are independent of such changes in prevalence of disease. Suppose we test a population of 100,000 persons in which 1% have the condition of interest (Fig. 7). The left-hand two cells will contain a total of 1000 individuals and the right-hand two cells will contain a total of 99,000. If, at the decision level chosen, the test is able to correctly identify 98% of affected individuals, then (0.98)(1000) or 980 will be true positives and 20 will be false negatives. The sensitivity of the test is 98%. If the prevalence were 10% instead of 1% (Fig. 8), the left-hand two cells would contain 10,000 individuals instead of 1000. The same test will still identify 98% of affected individuals correctly (if the decision level and disease spectrum have not changed); thus (0.98)(10,000) or 9800 would be true positives and 200 would be false positives. The sensitivity is still 98%; the total numbers change, but not the proportions of cases detected.[1]

[1]When extrapolating test performance data (sensitivity and specificity) obtained in one population to another population with a different prevalence of disease, one should consider whether the change in prevalence might be accompanied by a change in the spectrum of the disease, in which case the sensitivity of the test might be different in the second population. For example, if a test to detect cancer of the uterine cervix were evaluated in a population with a high prevalence that had not received Papanicolaou screening, a number of advanced cases would be found. On the other hand, a different population which received frequent and regular Papanicolaou screening might have not only a lower prevalence but also a different mix of cases, with a smaller proportion of advanced disease. Thus the sensitivity obtained in the first population might not be maintained in the second population, in which the spectrum of disease was shifted toward milder cases.

```
                             Disease or Condition

                           present              absent


                 "positive"      9800            18,000
         Test
         Result
                 "negative"       200            72,000


                 Total subjects = 100,000

                 Prevalence = 10%

                 Sensitivity = 98%

                 Specificity = 80%

                 PV(+) =         980        X 100 = 35.3%
                           9800 + 18,000
```

Figure 8. Four-cell matrix for hypothetical test as in Fig. 7, but with a prevalence of 10% instead of 1%.

On the other hand, let us look at predictive value. With a prevalence of 1%, a sensitivity of 0.98, and a specificity of 0.80, there are 980 true positives and 19,800 false positives (Fig. 7). The predictive value of a positive result is the fraction of positive test results which are true positives, or 980/(19,800 + 980) = 0.047. This is rather low because the false positive rate is high compared to the prevalence, resulting in many more false positive results (19,800) than true positive results (980). If the prevalence were 10% instead of 1% (Fig. 8), the predictive value of a positive test result would rise to 9800/(9800 + 18,000) = 0.353. While the false positive rate is still 20% (because the specificity does not change), the number of true positives has risen tenfold from 900 to 9000 because of the rise in prevalence of the disease. Now about one-third of all positive results are true positives.

Efficiency is defined as the fraction of results that are correct, that is, true positives and true negatives divided by all results. It is a combination of the predictive value of a positive result, TP/(TP + FP), and the predictive value of a negative result, TN/(TN + FN). It is dependent, then, on the sum of the diagonal boxes labeled TP and TN in Fig. 6. When disease prevalence is low and specificity is high, the TN box is quite large compared to all others. As a result, the predictive value of a negative result is very high and efficiency is usually high as well. This may be misleading, because in spite of the high calculated efficiency and predictive value of a negative result (due to the large TN), the sensitivity and/or the predictive value of a positive result may actually still be quite low. Thus, efficiency by itself is inadequate for judging test performance. Figure 9 illustrates such a situation in screening for an important but low-prevalence disease, phenylketonuria, which has a prevalence of 1 in 14,000 births. In this case a test with a specificity of 99% and a sensitivity of 29% would have a predictive value for negative results of 99.995% and an efficiency greater than 98.99%. Despite the impressive predictive value and efficiency, 71% of the actual cases would be missed, since the sensitivity is only 29%!

Sensitivity and specificity tell us about the probability that the test can detect the presence or absence of a condition in an individual. This helps us decide how well each test can do the job of ruling a condition in or out and thus also helps us decide which tests to order. Sensitivity and specificity are intrinsic fundamental properties of a test.

Predictive value and efficiency, on the other hand, are not intrinsic properties of a test. They derive from the interaction of sensitivity and specificity with prevalence. For each possible decision level, the corresponding sensitivity and specificity in combination with the prevalence control or determine a predictive value and efficiency. Each test, then, has a spectrum of predictive values and efficiencies, just as it has a spectrum of sensitivities and specificities. The predictive value and efficiency help us to understand the likelihood that a given result which we have obtained is a true result. Unfortunately, even this information is a gross oversimplification because all "positive" results are treated the same, that is, given the same weight. If the decision level for a test is 15 units and if the predictive value of a positive result is 90%, this suggests that a positive result (15

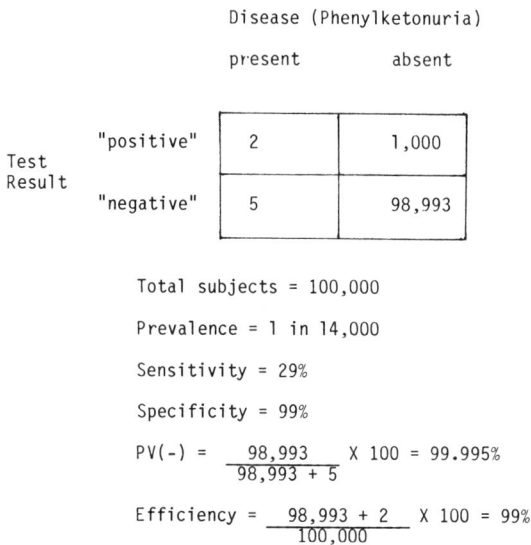

Disease (Phenylketonuria)

		present	absent
	"positive"	2	1,000
Test Result			
	"negative"	5	98,993

Total subjects = 100,000

Prevalence = 1 in 14,000

Sensitivity = 29%

Specificity = 99%

$$PV(-) = \frac{98,993}{98,993 + 5} \times 100 = 99.995\%$$

$$Efficiency = \frac{98,993 + 2}{100,000} \times 100 = 99\%$$

Figure 9. Four-cell matrix for a hypothetical test for phenylketonuria.

units or greater) has a 90% likelihood of being a true positive rather than a false positive. However, a result of 25 units probably is more likely to be a true positive than is a result of 16 units. Yet the predictive value concept treats all positives as if they have one single likelihood of being correct. What really is needed is a predictive value for each positive result: 16, 17, 18, . . . , that is, an expression of the likelihood of any individual value being truly positive (or negative). For this reason, expressing predictive value as a single fraction or percentage is an oversimplification by treating all positives as if they are the same and have identical likelihoods of being true positives. The consequences of this oversimplification is that we are led to have undue confidence in borderline results. We are led to believe that a result of 16 has a 90% likelihood of being a true positive. The 90% was calculated from all the positives, not just the borderline ones, and so is an average. In fact, 16 may have a rather low likelihood of being a true positive, particularly if 16 is frequently obtained from unaffected individuals (false positives). For these reasons, predictive values and efficiency have limited value and should be regarded only as a rough estimation of the likely significance of a given test result (using one particular decision level), not intrinsic or fundamental parameters of test performance.

III. CHOOSING DECISION LEVELS TO MINIMIZE COSTS

When an imperfect test is applied to a group of patients, some patients will be misclassified on the basis of the test results. These errors are potentially costly, since they may lead to a delay in instituting needed therapy (in the case of a false negative result) or unnecessary treatment, anxiety, and expense (in the case of a false positive result). If the actual—or even the relative—costs of false negative and false positive decisions can be stated, the relative total cost of all the incorrect decisions associated with a particular decision level can be estimated by using the TP and FP rates and the prevalence of the disease: (1) prevalence (PREV) indicates the proportion of subjects in the population studied who actually have the disease; (2) the FN rate (1.0 − TP rate) indicates the proportion of subjects who actually do have the disease but who will nonetheless be falsely diagnosed as negative by the test; (3) (PREV) × (FN rate) indicates the proportion of all subjects tested who will be incorrectly classified as not having the disease. These are the patients for whom the test makes falsely negative decisions. Thus, the cost due to false negative decisions is given by

$$(PREV) \times (FN \; rate) \times (cost \; of \; an \; FN \; decision)$$

Similarly, for false positive results: (1) (1.00 − PREV) indicates the proportion of subjects who do not have the disease; (2) the FP rate indicates the

proportion of subjects who do not have the disease but who will nonetheless have
a positive test result; (3) $(1.00 - PREV) \times$ (FP rate) indicates the proportion of
all subjects tested who will be incorrectly classified as having the disease. These
cases represent the falsely positive decisions. Thus, the cost due to false positive
decisions is given by

$$(1.00 - PREV) \times (FP \text{ rate}) \times (\text{cost of an FP decision})$$

Because each decision level is associated with a particular pair of TP and FP
rates, the total cost of the false positive and false negative misclassifications can
be calculated for every decision level. Unfortunately, decision level changes that
decrease the number of false negatives tend to increase the number of false
positives and vice versa. Changes in either sensitivity or specificity result in the
other member moving in the opposite direction. This cost trade-off is inherent in
all but perfect tests. The question is where the least costly balance occurs. By
plotting the total cost of misclassification (including both false positives and false
negatives) versus the decision level, the least costly decision levels can be
identified.

Note that, for a given test, changing the clinical application may result in a
different disease prevalence, a different set of costs, and even a different ROC
curve. This necessitates another calculation to find the optimal decision level for

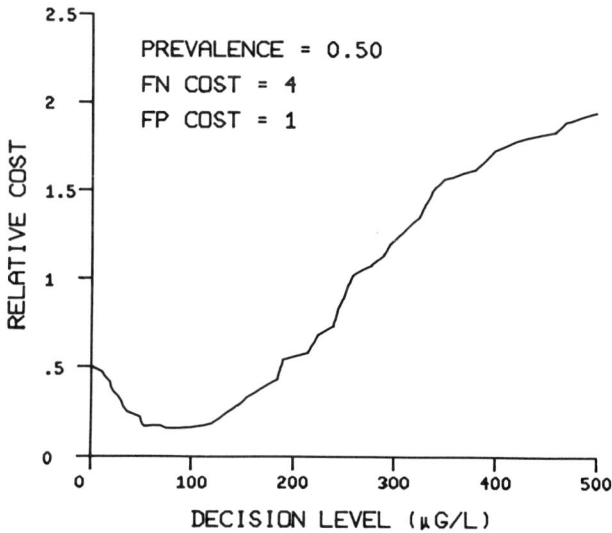

Figure 10. Relative cost of incorrect diagnoses as a function of the decision level chosen when
using myoglobin to identify patients with a myocardial infarct 5 h after the onset of chest pain. It is
assumed that the prevalence of infarctions is 50% and that the cost of a false negative (FN) result is
four times as great as the cost of a false positive (FP) result.

this alternative application. For example, the prevalence of acute myocardial infarction (AMI) in emergency room patients is different from the prevalence in hospitalized patients having cardiac surgery. The costs of false decisions may be different as well. Even the position of the ROC curve itself may change, (e.g., there may be more enzyme elevations in uninfarcted surgical patients because of surgical trauma to the skeletal and cardiac muscle). Thus, the optimal decision levels could be substantially different.

Consider the problem of diagnosing AMI in patients admitted to a coronary care unit (CCU) with chest pain. Suppose that, in this population, the prevalence of AMI is 50% and that, in this clinical situation, the cost of false negative results is four times as great as the cost of false positive results. The relative cost for each decision level can then be calculated, based on the corresponding true and false positive rates. Figure 10 is a plot of this relative cost versus the decision level for myoglobin at 5 h after the onset of pain. The relative cost is lowest (0.16) at a decision level of 76, corresponding to a TP rate of 0.97 and an FP rate of 0.20. This cost was calculated as described above from the prevalence (0.50), the cost of a false negative (4), the cost of a false positive (1), and the FN rate $(1.00 - \text{TP rate} = 1.00 - 0.97 = 0.03)$ and FP rate (0.20) at that decision level:

$$
\begin{aligned}
\text{Relative cost} =\ & (\text{PREV of AMI}) \times (\text{FN rate}) \times (\text{cost of an FN decision}) \\
& + (1.00 - \text{PREV}) \times (\text{FP rate}) \times (\text{cost of an FP decision}) \\
=\ & (0.50)(0.03)(4) + (0.50)(0.20)(1) \\
=\ & 0.16
\end{aligned}
$$

Looking at it somewhat differently (less quantitatively), suppose the goal were to confidently rule out AMI shortly after the onset of chest pain so that some patients could be transferred out of the coronary care unit. Assume that the cost of a false negative is very high and that early transfer of some patients is desirable to control CCU costs. Raising the targeted TP rate to 99% would make the false negative rate approach zero. (This would result in an increase in false positives since the decision level would have to be decreased.) Then if a patient had a negative result, it would be relatively certain that it was a true negative, not a false negative. Thus some, but not all, non-AMI subjects could be identified early in their course and could possibly be transferred out of the CCU. Dangerous false negatives would be minimized, while false positives (which are inconvenient but not dangerous) would be allowed to increase.

IV. RELATION OF NEW TESTS TO EXISTING TESTS

When a new test is ready to be introduced into routine usage—after its performance has been established and a decision level has been selected—it is important to consider how it is related to existing tests or procedures. This is, in fact, an issue which is ideally addressed at the beginning of the evaluation when framing the clinical question. Does the new test provide unique clinical information which complements the other data available? If so, then the new test can be added without replacing other tests or procedures. However, if the new test merely provides the same information as the existing tests but happens to be less invasive, less uncomfortable, less expensive, more convenient, more accurate, and so forth, then the "replaced" tests should actually be deleted from use in that setting. Often, new tests are added on without considering what data are redundant. This can lead to a false sense of confidence in the data. If new tests providing the same or similiar clinical information are added from time to time, there will be the false appearance of corroboration among independent parameters. If five tests used for establishing the diagnosis of acute myocardial infarction are all "positive," we are likely to feel more confidence in the diagnosis than if ony two or three or four are positive. This is reasonable if these are truly independent and unique parameters, but if they are all actually related and provide similar information, the additional confidence we have is not justified. We will have redundant information, wasted resources, and perhaps reach inappropriate conclusions about the significance of the results.

Some tests are helpful when other data have failed to answer the clinical question, or when other data have narrowed the possibilities to some degree. For example, lack of vitamin B_{12} or folate results in an increase in the size of the individual red blood cells, whereas most other causes of anemia result in red cells with normal or decreased volume. Thus the measurement of serum B_{12} is key in patients with macrocytic anemias but is unlikely to provide clinically useful information in patients with microcytic anemias. In such situations, the test should not be ordered initially, but should be ordered when the situation arises in which the test can make its unique contribution.

In summary, when implementing a test we should bear in mind its role and either add the test, substitute the test for others, or reserve it for special circumstances according to the actual findings of the evaluation.

V. A WORD ABOUT NORMAL RANGES

In this chapter, we have written relatively little about normal ranges, referent values and so forth and have not described how to establish conventional normal ranges. This is because for tests with relatively specific applications (diagnosis and/or monitoring of tumors, assessment of coronary artery disease or risk, diagnosis of myocardial infarction, assessment of fetal lung maturity), normal ranges derived from healthy volunteers or blood donors or laboratory workers are not appropriate. There is no necessary correspondence between the traditional "upper level of normal" (the 97.5 percentile of values from healthy volunteers) and the decision level which best separates patients into clinically important management subgroups. We need decision levels carefully selected to optimize the specific clinical distinction required for patient management.

For tests involving analytes under close homeostatic control (such as glucose, electrolytes, calcium, and hemoglobin) which are widely used to screen ambulatory patients, normal ranges based on typical values found in healthy controls have traditionally been used. Although the presence of an abnormal value for such a test is often thought to imply some sort of physiological abnormality, the clinical importance of mildly "abnormal" results in asymptomatic patients is often unclear. For patient management, the value at which the risks of nonintervention exceed the risks of intervention is more important than the point at which results become "abnormal" by the arbitrary standard of the 97.5 percentile of the "normal population." In practice, clinicians often have their own "action points" which do not correspond to the traditional normal range.

VI. SUMMARY

The first step in designing a study to evaluate the clinical usefulness of a test is to establish clearly and explicitly the clinical goal. It is essential to identify what issue of consequence to patient management is to be addressed by the test. We suggest the following guidelines for a clinical test evaluation or diagnostic trial: (1) Choose study subjects who are representative of the clinical population to which the test is ultimately to be applied. (2) Perform all tests being evaluated on all the subjects; perform all tests on an individual subject at the same point in the subject's clinical course. (3) Classify the subjects as affected versus unaffected or diseased versus nondiseased by rigorous and complete means so that the true diagnoses or outcomes are approached closely. Diagnostic maneuvers going beyond routine clinical practice may be required for the purpose of the evaluation. All diagnostic criteria should be independent of the test or tests being studied. (4) Evaluate and compare test performance at all decision levels by using ROC curves. (5) Select decision levels for the test(s) being evaluated based on the ROC curve, the intended use of the test, the prevalence of the condition, and the relative costs of false positive and false negative results.

VII. ILLUSTRATIVE EXAMPLE: APOLIPOPROTEIN A-I

Persons with signs and symptoms of coronary artery disease (CAD) are often considered by their physicians to be candidates for coronary artery angiography. The angiographic procedure is performed with the expectation that the findings will influence the management of these individuals. For example, in some fraction the angiography will reveal obstructive lesions of a nature indicating that coronary bypass surgery would be a relevant management alternative. However, not all persons undergoing coronary angiography have sufficient disease to indicate a surgical or other aggressive intervention. It would be valuable, then, to have an inexpensive, noninvasive, safe means (serum assay) of identifying some or all of those individuals who might otherwise undergo coronary angiography but who, in fact are very unlikely to exhibit clinically important coronary disease suitable for aggressive intervention. Such a means would permit screening of these people in order to eliminate angiography for some of them, resulting in fewer angiographic procedures and a savings in health care dollars.

The clinical question, then, would be: "Does this patient with clinical evidence of CAD who is a candidate for angiography have clinically important angiographically demonstrable coronary artery disease?" "Clinically important" would refer to those lesions which make the patient a candidate for some aggressive intervention. If we were to design a study to evaluate one or more tests which might be able to provide this clinically useful information, we would begin by identifying a sample population to test prospectively, such as 1000 consecutive patients with specified evidence of CAD who were referred by their physician for angiography. Before angiography, each subject would receive the battery of tests under evaluation. All subjects would ultimately be classified definitively on the basis of their angiographic findings without knowledge of the blood test results, all the angiographic data being reviewed and interpreted by more than one person. Once the subjects have been classified as having or not having clinically important disease, the sensitivities and specificities achievable by each blood test under study would be examined with ROC curves. If one or more tests displayed good performance—had good ROC curves—we would go on to determine the optimal decision level and determine what ultimate gains we realize by using the test(s).

We choose this example because a study similar to this was recently published (Maciejko et al., 1983). Let us examine what was done and what was learned from the study. The study group comprised 108 male patients with chest pain or suspected CAD or both who were going to have diagnostic coronary angiography. Blood lipids as well as apolipoprotein A-I by an RIA were measured. Angiograms were reviewed without prior knowledge of the serum lipid or lipoprotein results. On the basis of the angiograms, 25 did not have clinically important lesions (stenosis of greater than 50% of at least one vessel). Eighty-three had single-, double-, or triple- vessel disease. ROC curves analysis of the raw data presented in the paper showed clearly that apolipoprotein A-I was quite effective at distinguishing between the 25 persons without clinically important CAD and the 83 who did have clinically important CAD. There was little overlap in the results from the two subgroups. Furthermore, ROC curve analysis showed that high-density lipoprotein (HDL)–cholesterol was rather poor at classifying the subgroups and clearly inferior to apolipoprotein A-I.

Unfortunately, a study population of 108 is small and limits the resolution of the ROC curve and the certainty with which we can estimate the actual performance parameters and the decision levels corresponding to any particular sensitivity or specificity. We can see from the data in that paper something of the value of applying the test, but it is difficult to establish this with confidence. To use the test, we must select a decision level. We could estimate relative costs of false positives (persons without important lesions who nonetheless have "positive" results and thus would undergo angiography) and false negatives (persons with clinically important lesions but negative results who are incorrectly denied angiography and perhaps beneficial intervention). We could then find the decision level with the lowest relative cost as described in the text earlier. This decision level would be optimized for this specific purpose, that is, deciding who with clinical symptoms of CAD might benefit from angiography. It would not be appropriate to use this decision level to screen apparently healthy persons for occult CAD, or to screen 35-year-old persons who want to start jogging 50 miles a week, or to predict who would do well following coronary artery bypass surgery. The test might be helpful in those situations, but a separate study is required to determine the test's performance in each of those circumstances and to choose specific decision levels if, indeed, the test is effective for answering any of those other questions.

APPENDIX: PREPARATION OF ROC CURVES

A plot of the receiver operating characteristic curve provides a graphic display of the relationship between the true positive and false positive rates of a test as the decision level is varied.

The accompanying table (Table I) illustrates the steps involved in constructing an ROC curve from the data obtained in a clinical test evaluation.

1. Arrange the combined test results (from both the affected and unaffected groups) in a single list in descending order (column A).

2. Copy the results from the affected group to column B and the results from the unaffected group to column F.

3. Assign ranks to the values in the affected group, giving the largest value a rank of 1 (column C). If two or more subjects in the group have identical values, assign each of the identical values the average of the ranks that the identical values would have received had they been slightly different from each other. For example, in column B the 5th and 6th values are identical (85). If these values had been 84.99 and 85.01, they would have received ranks 5 and 6. Since the recorded values are identical, each is assigned the average rank of 5.5: $(5 + 6)/2 = 5.5$.

4. Convert the ranks in column C to true positive percentiles (column D) using the formula

$$p = [r/(n + 1)] \times 100$$

where p is the percentile, r the rank, and n the total number of results in the group.

Table I. Raw and Calculated Data for Preparing ROC Curves

A All results (concentration units)	B Results for affected group	C Ranks for affected group	D True positive percentiles for affected group	E Interpolated true positive percentiles	F Results for unaffected group	G Ranks for unaffected group	H False positive percentiles for affected group	I Interpolated false positive percentiles
150	150	1	10	—	—	—	—	—
120	120	2	20	—	—	—	—	—
105	—	—	—	27.5	105	1	10	—
100	100	3	30	—	—	—	—	13
90	90	4	40	—	—	—	—	19
88	—	—	—	46	88	2	20	—
85	85	5.5	55	—	—	—	—	25
85	85	5.5	55	—	—	—	—	25
82	—	—	—	64	82	3	30	—
80	80	7	70	—	—	—	—	31
70	70	8	80	—	—	—	—	34
50	50	9	90	—	—	—	—	40
50	—	—	—	—	50	4	40	—
45	—	—	—	—	45	5	50	—
40	—	—	—	—	40	6	60	—
35	—	—	—	—	35	7	70	—
25	—	—	—	—	25	8	80	—
15	—	—	—	—	15	9	90	—

For example, the 4th result in the group of the nine affected subjects would have a percentile

$$p = [4/(9 + 1)] \times 100 = 40$$

5. For results in the unaffected group in column F) which fall between pairs of adjoining results in the affected group, true positive percentiles[2] are calculated by interpolation (column E), using the formula

$$P = P_A + (P_B - P_A) \times (R_A - R)/(R_A - R_B)$$

where P is the percentile to be calculated by interpolation, P_A the percentile on the line just above the desired percentile, P_B the percentile on the line just below the desired percentile, R the result for which the percentile is to be calculated by interpolation, R_A the result from the line just above the desired percentile, and R_B the result from the line just below the desired percentile.

For example, in column F there is a result of 88 for a patient in the unaffected group. This value falls between results of 90 and 85 in the affected group in column B. Thus, a true positive percentile must be interpolated.

$$
\begin{aligned}
P_A &= 40 \ \text{(column D)} \\
P_B &= 55 \ \text{(column D)} \\
R &= 88 \ \text{(column F)} \\
R_A &= 90 \ \text{(column B)} \\
R_B &= 85 \ \text{(column B)}
\end{aligned}
$$

Thus,

$$
\begin{aligned}
P &= 40 + (55 - 40) \times (90 - 88)/(90 - 85) \\
&= 40 + 6 \\
&= 46
\end{aligned}
$$

This interpolated true positive percentile of 46 is recorded in column E.

The operations in steps 3 through 5 are now carried out for the results from the unaffected group:

6. Assign ranks to the results in column F from the unaffected group, recording the ranks in column G. (Treat ties according to the procedure described in step 3.)

7. Convert the ranks in column G to false positive percentiles in column H using the formula $p = [r/(n + 1)] \times 100$.

8. For results in the affected group (column B) which fall between pairs of adjacent values in the unaffected group (column F), calculate false positive percentiles by inter-

---

[2]At a decision level of 105, there is a false positive percentile in column H derived from the results and ranks observed for the unaffected group (columns F and G). However, because there were no observations at 105 from the affected group, there is not a true positive percentile entered in column D. The ROC curve comprises true positive–false positive percentile pairs. To plot the ROC curve, then, for the decision level 105, the true positive percentile must be interpolated from the data in column D and then entered into column E.

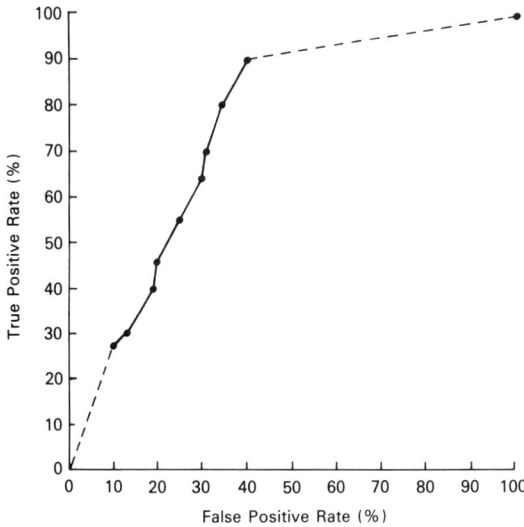

Figure 11. ROC curve for data in Table I. The solid portion represents the true and false positive rates from the range where results from the affected and unaffected groups overlap. The dashed portion represents extension of the ROC curve to the (0, 0) point, where all results are below the decision level, and to the (100, 100) point, where all results are above the decision level.

polation, using the procedure outlined in step 5. Record the interpolated percentiles in column I.

9. An ROC curve for the region where results from the affected and unaffected groups overlap (results 50–105) can now be constructed by plotting the true positive percentiles (in columns D and E) on the vertical axis against the false positive percentiles (in column H and I) on the horizontal axis. See Fig. 11.

The ROC curve shows the relation between the true positive and false positive rates in the range where results from the affected and unaffected groups overlap (see solid portion of curve in Fig. 11). The shape of the ROC curve beyond the highest result for the unaffected group and beyond the lowest result for the affected group cannot be determined from the data in the sample. The following reasoning is sometimes used to extend the ROC curve to the (0, 0) and (100, 100) points: If the decision level is lowered sufficiently, all results (from both affected and unaffected subjects) will be above the decision level, yielding a true positive rate of 100% and a false positive rate of 100%. Thus the ROC curve must pass through the (100, 100) point. Similarly, if the decision level is raised sufficiently, both the true and false positive rates will fall to zero; thus the ROC curve must pass through the (0, 0) point. These extended portions of the ROC curve are indicated by dashed lines in Fig. 11 to indicate that for these portions of the curve the starting and ending points are known, but the actual shape is not.

In assessing the results of test evaluation studies, including ROC curves, the statistical

126
Mark H. Zweig and E. Arthur Robertson

uncertainty of percentages estimated from small samples should be kept in mind. For example, if on the basis of a random sample of 100 patients, 10% are found to have a test result greater than, say, 50 units, the 95% confidence limits for the true proportion of the population of similar patients having a result greater than 50 units are 5–18%. If the 10% proportion were estimated on the basis of a sample of only 10 patients, the confidence limits would range from <1 to 46% (Clopper and Pearson, 1934).

REFERENCES

Beck, J. R. (1982). Quantitative logic and new diagnostic tests. *Arch. Intern. Med.* **142**, 681–682.
Clopper, C. J., and Pearson, E. S. (1934). The use of confidence or fiducial limits illustrated in the case of binomial. *Biometrika* **26**, 404–413.
Kassirer, J. P., and Pauker, S. G. (1978). Should diagnostic testing be regulated? *N. Engl. J. Med.* **299**, 947–949.
Lufkin, E. G., DeRemee, R. A., and Rohrbach, M. S. (1983). The predictive value of serum angiotensin-converting enzyme activity in the differential diagnosis of hypercalcemia. *Mayo Clin. Proc.* **58**, 447–451.
Maciejko, J. J., Holmes, D. R., Kottke, B. A., Zinsmeister, A. R., Dinh, D. M., and Mao, S. J. T. (1983). Apolipoprotein A-I as a marker of angiographically assessed coronary-artery disease. *N. Engl. J. Med.* **309**, 385–389.
Ransohoff, D. F., and Feinstein, A. R. (1978). Problems of spectrum and bias in evaluating the efficacy of diagnostic tests. *N. Eng. J. Med.* **299**, 926–930.
Van Steirteghem, C. A., Zweig, M. H., Robertson, E. A., Bernard, R. M., Putzeys, G. A., and Bieva, C. J. (1982). Comparison of the effectiveness of four clinical chemical assays in classifying patients with chest pain. *Clin. Chem.* **28**, 1319–1324.
Zweig, M. H., and Robertson, E. A. (1982). Why we need better test evaluations. *Clin. Chem.* **28**, 1272–1276.

SELECTED LITERATURE

Beck, J. R. and Shultz, E. K. (1986). The use of relative operating characteristic (ROC) curves in test performance evaluation. *Arch. Pathol. Lab. Med.* **110**, 13–20.
Benson, E. S., Connelly, D. P., and Burke, M. D. (1982). Symposium on Test Selection Strategies. *Clin. Lab. Med.* **2**, 683–901.
Gerhardt, W. and Keller, H. (1985). Evaluation of test data from clinical studies. *Scand. J. Clin. Lab. Invest.* **46**, Suppl. 181, 1–74.
Griner, P. F., Mayewski, R. J., Mushlin, A. I., and Greenland, P. (1981). Selection and interpretation of diagnostic tests and procedures. Principles and applications. *Ann. Intern. Med.* **94**, 553–587.
Griner, P. F., and Glaser, R. J. (1982). Misuse of laboratory tests and diagnostic procedures. *N. Engl. J. Med.* **307**, 1336–1339.
Jacquez, J. A., ed. (1972). "Computer Diagnosis and Diagnostic Methods," pp. 8–44. Charles C. Thomas, Springfield, Illinois.
McMaster University Department of Clinical Epidemiology and Biostatistics. (1981) How to read clinical journals: II. To learn about a diagnostic test. *Can. Med. Assoc. J.* **124**, 703–710.

McNeil, B. J., and Adelstein, S. J. (1976). Determining the value of diagnostic and screening tests. *J. Nucl. Med.* **17,** 439–448.

McNeil, B. J. and Hanley, J. A. (1984). Statistical approaches to the analysis of receiver operating characteristic (ROC) curves. *Medical Decision Making* **4,** 137–150.

McNeil, B. J., Keeler, E., and Adelstein, S. J. (1975). Primer on certain elements of medical decision making. *N. Engl. J. Med.* **293,** 211–215.

Metz, C. E. (1978). Basic principles of ROC analysis. *Semin. Nucl. Med.* **8,** 283–298.

Ransohoff, D. F. and Feinstein, A. R. (1978). Problems of spectrum and bias in evaluating the efficacy of diagnostic tests. *N. Engl. J. Med.* **299,** 926–930.

Reuben, D. B. (1984). Learning diagnostic restraint. *N. Engl. J. Med.* **310,** 591–593.

Riegelman, R. K. (1981). "Studying a Study and Testing a Test. How to Read the Medical Literature." Little, Brown, Boston.

Robertson, E. A., and Zweig, M. H. (1981). Use of receiver operating characteristic curves to evaluate the clinical performance of analytical systems. *Clin. Chem.* **27,** 1569–1574.

Robertson, E. A., Zweig, M. H., and Van Steirteghem, A. C. (1983). Evaluating the clinical efficacy of laboratory tests. *Am. J. Clin. Pathol.* **79,** 78–86.

Turner, D. A. (1978). An intuitive approach to receiver operating characteristic curve analysis. *J. Nucl. Med.* **19,** 213–220.

Weinstein, M. C., and Fineberg, H. V., eds. (1980). "Clinical Decision Analysis," pp. 75–130. Saunders, Philadelphia.

Chapter 5

Data Reduction Techniques
for Immunoassay

George F. Johnson

Department of Pathology
University of Iowa
Iowa City, Iowa 52242

I. PURPOSE OF CHAPTER

The goal of this chapter is to present the important ideas needed to understand calibration methods in immunoassay. The viewpoint is that of a user of automated data reduction techniques. By removing some of the mystery behind microcomputer data reduction packages, the laboratory worker can make better decisions about which particular data reduction technique is suitable for each immunoassay.

II. INTRODUCTION

Almost all high-volume assays in clinical chemistry use automated result calculation. Older manual data reduction methods required that pencil and graph paper be used to interpolate assay results from a hand-drawn standard curve. Assay response versus concentration curves were generated either by drawing straight lines between adjacent points or by "fitting" a "best line," either straight or nonlinear, by eye. Errors could be made in plotting the points, and considerable variation between individuals could be found in fitting the same data points. Errors of interpolation from the standard curve were common. The results of quality control samples also were subject to bias since the analyst did not read these results blindly from the calibration curve and already knew the usual value for these samples. As in all paper-and-pencil systems, transcription errors were common.

In contrast, automated calibration procedures increase productivity by eliminating the tedious manual interpolation process, eliminating observer bias in reading quality control values, and decreasing the occurrence of transcription errors. Thus, in any analytical chemistry system, immediate benefits can be obtained by automating the results calculation process.

I will outline in this chapter the two main approaches to a calibration process in immunoassay: (1) interpolation and (2) the use of a model. The interpolation approach simply connects mathematical curves from one calibration point to the next with the implicit assumption that the points are without experimental error or that the error is very small. The model approach is based on the assumption that a mathematical curve would exactly describe the immunoassay data if there were no experimental errors. The curve does not pass exactly through all the calibration points that describe the analytical response versus concentration plot. The model has adjustable parameters which are varied by mathematical software to generate a curve that passes "close" to the experimental calibration points. I will also discuss how the immunoassay data reduction method can be used to learn more about the performance characteristics of an immunoassay and its quality control.

III. INTERPOLATION TECHNIQUES
OF DATA REDUCTION

The simplest interpolation technique is by linear segments between concentration points. This approach is shown in Fig. 1. If r_1 and r_2 are the analytical

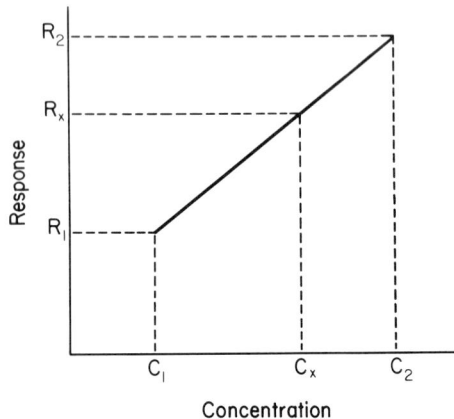

Figure 1. Simple linear interpolation.

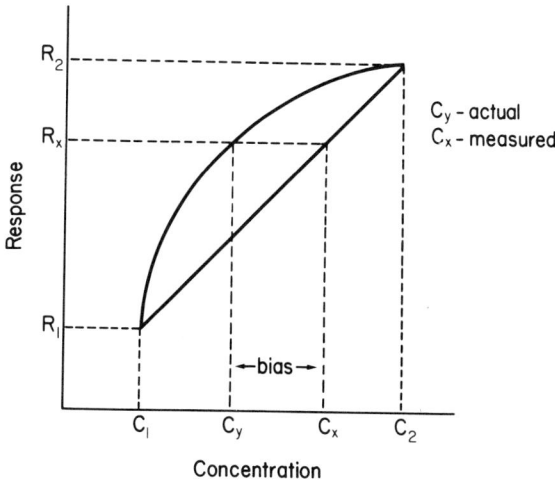

Figure 2. Bias in linear interpolation.

responses at concentrations c_1 and c_2, then a response observed between r_1 and r_2 designated as r_x can be converted to concentration c_x from the proportionality shown in Eq. (1).

$$\frac{c_x - c_1}{c_2 - c_1} = \frac{r_x - r_1}{r_2 - r_1} \tag{1}$$

Solving for c_x in Eq. (1), we derive the linear interpolation formula shown in Eq. (2).

$$c_x = c_1 + \frac{r_x - r_1}{r_2 - r_1}(c_2 - c_1) \tag{2}$$

Equation (2) is valid for either $r_2 > r_1$ or $r_1 > r_2$. Linear interpolation can easily be programmed on a microcomputer and automates the tedious, error-prone manual technique of reading the unknown concentration from graph paper.

   This simple technique also illustrates well the potential disadvantages of interpolation methods for data reduction. As can be seen in Fig. 2, if the curved line represents the real change in response between c_1 and c_2 then the linear approximation will yield c_x, which is not identical with c_y, the correct concentration for response r_x. This means that c_x, the concentration from the linear approximation, will be biased to some unknown extent. Bias can be reduced in linear interpolation by making transformations. For instance, if response versus the logarithm of concentration were approximately linear then we would substitute the logarithm of concentration for concentration in Eq. (2) and take the antilog after interpolation to determine concentration. Such a scheme is limited only by the number of different transformations of r and c that can be imagined.

Another approach is to use a higher-order interpolating polynomial. Instead of the simple straight line ($y = ax + b$), a third-order polynomial (cubic) can be used ($y = a + bx + cx^2 + dx^3$). This procedure is commonly called the method of cubic splines. A different third-order polynomial is used between each pair of points in the standard curve. The collection of polynomials go through all the points and the resulting curve is smooth to the eye. The smoothness is a result of equal slopes when two polynomials meet at a point. A second condition is that rates of change of the slopes are also equal at each point. In more mathematical language we say that when two polynomials meet at a point the first and second derivatives of the two curves are equal.

The final condition involves the two end points of the calibration curve. If we require known fixed slopes at these points, the resulting spline is called a bound spline, and if we require only that the second derivatives be equal to zero, the curve is called a natural spline (Burden *et al.*, 1978). Because of the smoothness of the spline, we can remove much of the bias shown in Fig. 2 by the abrupt change in slope in the linear point-to-point interpolation.

IV. MODELS AND STATISTICAL APPROACHES TO DATA REDUCTION

A. Statistical Error

Figure 3 shows the type of curve that we might expect from a competitive immunoassay, where the response variable could be either radioactive counts or enzyme activity. The data points are what we actually observe and the continu-

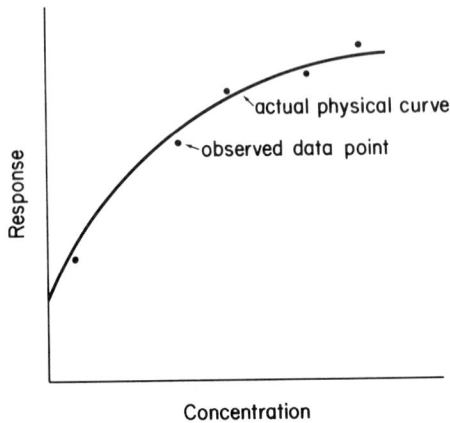

Figure 3. Immunoassay calibration curve.

ous curve is a representation of the underlying physical process that relates analytical response and concentration. As can be seen, even if the actual relationship were given to us as an equation, our experimental points would not fall exactly on the curve but, on the average, would cluster close to the curve. This is because of the random experimental errors made during the immunoassay; these include pipetting errors, variable separation of free and bound ligand, and random errors made in the analytical response. These errors are all of a statistical nature and are present in all analytical systems whether manual or automated.

B. Fitting Models to Data

The mathematical relationship between analytical response and concentration is called a *model*. For many analytes measured spectrophotometrically in clinical chemistry, we know that absorbance measured after a chemical reaction is directly proportional to analyte concentration. We construct a standard curve using a linear model whose *parameters* are the slope and intercept. While we know that the relationship between analytical response and concentration is linear, the actual parameters (slope and intercept) of the standard curve must be determined from the data obtained by observing the analytical response from known standard concentrations. If we run only one standard and assume the intercept to be equal to zero, the calculation of the one parameter in the model is obvious. However, if we run six standards of different concentrations, a straight line must be fit by eye or by a mathematical calculation. The parameters of the model are adjusted so that what the model predicts is close to what is observed. The criterion used for closeness of fit determines how we mathematically fit the model.

C. Least Squares

The most common approach to fitting models to data is the method of least squares. The example of the straight line is shown in Fig. 4. The vertical distance is shown between the measured response variable (y) and what the model would predict at that value of concentration (x) given fixed values for the two parameters. As we vary the parameters of the model, the vertical distances will also vary. The optimal set of parameters are those which minimize the sum of the squares of all the vertical distances. If each point in the standard curve is designated as (x_i, y_i), where the subscript i varies from 1 to n, the vertical distance (d_i) associated with each point can be written as $y_i - \hat{y}_i$ where $\hat{y}_i$ is the predicted model value at x_i from the linear model equation $\hat{y}_i = \hat{m}x_i + \hat{b}$. The "hats" over m and b are used because we only *estimate* the unknown parameters of the model from the data. These estimates are derived by minimizing the sum of squares given in Eq. (3).

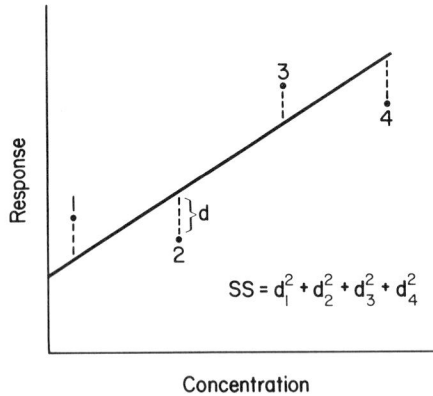

Figure 4. Straight-line fit by least squares.

$$\text{Sum of squares} = d_1^2 + d_2^2 + \cdots + d_i^2 + \cdots + d_n^2 = \sum_{i=1}^{n} d_i^2 \qquad (3)$$

The quality of the estimates depends on the inherent statistical noise at each point and the number of data points. The less the noise and the greater the number of points, the better are the estimates of the actual parameter values that define the model.

D. Nonlinear Least Squares

Both linear and nonlinear model parameters are common. The parameters a, b, c, and d that define the cubic polynomial $y = a + bx + cx^2 + dx^3$ are all linear even though y is a nonlinear function of the variable x; the parameters are linear because if any one is varied while the others and x are held fixed, a linear change in y is observed. In the model $y = a/(b + x)$, a is a linear parameter and b is a nonlinear parameter. Models in which all the parameters are linear can easily be handled mathematically: a numerical solution with a defined series of steps can be found for the least-squares parameter estimates.

Estimation of parameters in a nonlinear model requires a process of numerical *iteration*. This is a multistep numerical procedure where the parameter estimates are adjusted with each step, and when the minimum sum of squares is closely approximated, the process is said to have achieved *convergence*. Usually the criterion for convergence is a very small change in the parameter estimates from one iteration to the next, without *exceeding* a maximum number of iterations. Nonlinear models for immunoassay can now routinely be used in laboratories because of the rapid development, low cost and speed of the microcomputer system. Most commercial immunoassay systems offer both interpolation and model fitting software based on numerical least-squares procedures.

V. NONLINEAR MODELS IN IMMUNOASSAY

A. The Four-Parameter Logistic Model

The most often used nonlinear model in immunoassay is the four-parameter logistic model (Rodbard, 1974). It can be written in a variety of forms; a common form is shown in Eq. (4).

$$y = \frac{a-d}{1 + (x/c)^b} + d \qquad (4)$$

In this equation y is the analytical response and x is the concentration. When $x = 0$ the y intercept is a, and as x approaches infinity y approaches the asymptote d as shown in Fig. 5. Substitution of $x = c$ in the equation yields $y = (a + d)/2$, which is halfway between the intercept and the asymptote. This model has been successful in fitting a variety of immunoassays because it simulates the actual physical characteristics of immunoassay systems (Rodbard and McClean, 1977). As concentration increases, the antibody present becomes more saturated and the analytical response of counts or enzyme activity approaches a limiting value. The exponential term b allows the curve to deviate from the simple hyperbolic shape observed when $b = 1$. The model when $b = 1$ is the physical model one would expect from isotope dilution when antibody is used to sample an excess of mixed labeled ligand and unlabeled ligand that bind identically.

Until microcomputers became widely available, Eq. (4) was not fitted to data directly to estimate all four parameters, but a transformation of this equation was commonly used. A new variable Y is defined as $(y - d)/(a - d)$ and Eq. (5) can easily be derived from Eq. (4).

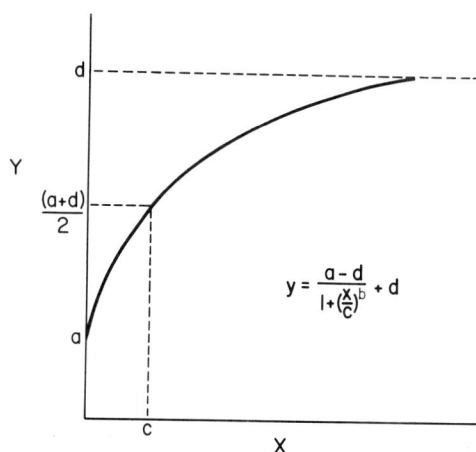

Figure 5. Graphic interpretation of the four parameters of the logistic equation.

$$\frac{Y}{1-Y} = \frac{1}{(x/c)^b} \qquad \text{where } Y = (y-d)/(a-d) \qquad (5)$$

By taking the natural logarithm of both sides of Eq. (5), the linear transformation shown in Eq. (6) is derived.

$$\text{logit}(Y) = \ln\left(\frac{Y}{1-Y}\right) = -\ln\left(\frac{x}{c}\right)^b = \ln c^b - b \ln x \qquad (6)$$

Before this linearized equation can be used, estimates of the parameters a and d must be obtained. Since a is the predicted analytical response at $x = 0$, the observed response at zero concentration is used. The parameter d is the limiting value of the analytical response (y) as concentration (x) approaches infinity. In radioimmunoassay where the bound fraction is counted, this is the nonspecific counts bound and can be estimated by including a tube with no antibody but with labeled ligand added. With commercial immunoassays, reagent systems are not always packaged so that d can easily be determined. If poor estimates of a and d are made, then Eq. (6) will not yield a linear transformation and the standard points, transformed to logit, will not fall on a straight line when plotted versus concentration. The nonlinearity which results when a poor estimate of d is used will produce bias in the results for unknowns read off this standard curve. In the next section, on the statistical variation associated with the measured response variable, it will be shown that transformation of the response variable illustrated by the linearized form of Eq. (6) also can greatly transform the statistical variation observed.

B. Noise about the Standard Curve

A measure of statistical variation of the response variable is the standard deviation of the estimate. This estimation of variance in the analytical response is calculated from the minimum sum of squares (SS_{min}) in the least-squares parameter estimation procedure and is given in Eq. (7).

$$SD_{est}^2 = SS_{min}/(n-p) \qquad (7)$$

The variable n in this equation is the number of data points in the standard curve and p is the number of parameters estimated. The SD_{est} will estimate experimental noise associated with the response variable if this noise is essentially constant at each response along the concentration axis. This is known as homogeneity of variance. When this condition holds, the SD_{est} would estimate the same quantity as obtained by assaying many standards at the same concentration value and calculating the observed standard deviation. The standard deviation of the response variable usually varies with the magnitude of the analytical response. One important contributing factor is the noise of volumetric measurements, and another is instrumental variation. In spectrophotometric measurements, as absorbance increases, so does spectrophotometric noise. When emission from radioisotopes is counted, the variance in counts measured is equal to the actual counts present. If there is substantial change in variance of the response variable as a function of concentration, the estimates of the parameters of the standard curve by least squares will be influenced. This is a consequence of the largest deviation having the most effect on parameter estimates. For all the points to contribute to the parameter estimates, the response variable must be weighted. For least squares this is accomplished as shown in Eq. (8).

$$SS = \sum_{i=1}^{n} w_i^2 (y_i - \hat{y}_i)^2 \tag{8}$$

The weighting factor is w_i, and when $w_i = 1$ we have ordinary unweighted least squares. The usual approach to weighting is to set $w_i = 1/\sigma_i$, where σ_i is the estimated standard deviation of the response variable y_i. The contribution of the noisier response values to the total sum of squares in Eq. (8) will, after weighting, be no more than that of any other point.

We can now comment on the effect of the linear transformation that gave the logit function of Eq. (6). Equation (9) shows the approximation used to estimate the effect of a transformation of the response variable on the variance.

$$\sigma_z^2 \cong \left| \frac{dz}{dy} \right|^2 \sigma_y^2 \tag{9}$$

If we set $z = \text{logit}(Y) = \ln[Y/(1 - Y)]$ and calculate the derivative and substitute into Eq. (9), we obtain the following result.

$$\sigma_z^2 \cong \frac{1}{Y^2(1-Y)^2} \sigma_y^2 \tag{10}$$

We can immediately see the huge multiplying effect on the variance (σ_z^2) when Y approaches 0 or approaches 1: small errors in these points would have an unduly large effect on the slope and intercept estimated for Eq. (6) from the data if the weighting factor $W_i^2 = 1/\sigma_z^2 = Y^2(1 - Y)^2/\sigma_y^2$ were not used (Rodbard, 1971). In practice, only the $Y^2(1 - Y)^2$ term is used since the change in variance over the nontransformed response variable is usually small.

The four-parameter logistic model [Eq. (6)] can be fit to data with appropriate weighting if the experimental data are available to calculate the weights. Software requires a weighting function that supplies the standard deviation (noise) in the response variable y given the numerical value of y. Most laboratories use software that fits Eq. (6) to data without the use of weighting because automated collection of replicate data to determine the statistical variation in the response variable as a function of its value is not available. How to obtain these data will be discussed in the next section.

C. Standard Deviation Estimates from Duplicates

Equation (11) gives the common formula for estimating the standard deviation of a variable y from replicate data: $\bar{y}$ in this formula is the mean of all the n values.

$$SD_n^2 = \sum_{i=1}^{n} (y_i - \bar{y})^2/(n - 1) \tag{11}$$

When only two data values y_1 and y_2 are known, Eq. (11) simplifies to Eq. (12).

$$SD_2^2 = (y_1 - y_2)^2/2 \tag{12}$$

If we pool all the data from N sets of duplicates, the average SD is determined by Eq. (13).

$$SD_N^2 = \sum_{i=1}^{N} (y_{1i} - y_{2i})^2/2N \tag{13}$$

The subscript i refers to the particular duplicate pair (y_{1i}, y_{2i}). Duplicate data can be combined from multiple standard curves to generate estimated standard deviations of the response value at each concentration value. Duplicate data can also be used from controls and patient samples. In this case, data are usually divided into ranges (bins) of the response variable and an SD is associated with the mean response in each range (Rodbard et al., 1976). For use in weighting, the standard deviation data can be fit by least squares to a straight line, quadratic equation, or other model. The variance model and its estimated parameters are then used to generate an expected weight (1/SD) for any value of the response variable (y) needed by the software for calibration model fitting. In automated nonisotopic immunoassay systems, replicate data are usually not available because of reagent cost, and unweighted calibration curves are used.

D. Within-Run Variation as a Function of Concentration

The standard deviation calculated from duplicates represents the within-run variation for the response variable. If this noise is reflected through the calibration curve, the expected within-run variation in concentration can be estimated. Equation (13) gives the standard deviation expected for one sample; the average of duplicates is usually reported, and this standard deviation is decreased by the factor of the square root of 2 when used with the average of duplicates. With competitive immunoassays, the slope of the response versus concentration curve continually decreases as concentration increases (Fig. 5). At a high concentration a small change in response produces a much larger change in concentration than the same response change at a lower concentration. The within-run standard deviation in concentration increases with absolute concentration. As as example, we can rearrange the four-parameter logistic formula [Eq. (6)] to solve for concentration as a function of the response variable as follows:

$$X = c \left(\frac{a - d}{y - d} - 1 \right)^{1/b} = c \left(\frac{a - y}{y - d} \right)^{1/b} \tag{14}$$

If we know the parameters of the model, then SD_x can be determined given SD_y. Equation (9) can be used as an approximation for this transformation as well.

$$SD_x^2 \cong \left| \frac{dx}{dy} \right|^2 SD_y^2 \tag{15}$$

Combining Eq. (15) and (14) gives the formula shown in Eq. (16).

$$SD_x \cong \left| \frac{[1 + (x/c)^b]^2 c^b}{(d - a)bx^{b-1}} \right| SD_y \tag{16}$$

This equation cannot be used at $x = 0$ but will give a reasonable estimate of the variation expected at higher concentrations. Knowledge of the expected coefficient of variation at a given concentration value can help determine the dynamic range that is acceptable from a standard curve before samples are diluted for reanalysis.

E. Number of Standards

The minimum number of standards that can be used in any clinical chemistry procedure is one, and even then a suitable blank is included to simulate a zero calibrator. When the calibration model is a straight line, two parameters (slope and intercept) must be estimated, and two points are required. Obviously, if a least-squares approach is used to fit a straight line to only two points, the line will go exactly through both points. This result is easily generalized and understood when higher-order polynomials are used. A quadratic polynomial has three parameters, and if three points are provided, a least-squares solution will go through all three points. A cubic polynomial has four parameters, and with four points in the standard curve, the least-squares solution of the four parameters would generate a polynomial that would pass through all four points. For nonlinear models, a similar phenomenon may also take place when the number of parameters equals the number of calibrator points. A minimum of one more calibrator than the number of parameters is required to escape almost "perfect fit" artifacts with least-squares numerical methods. In order that discrepant calibrator point can be dropped from a standard curve, a reasonable recommendation is that two more calibrator points be used than the number of parameters estimated; with this recommendation six standard curve points would be used with the four-parameter logistic model.

VI. SUMMARY

Both interpolative and model-based calibration methods are in wide use. Interpolative methods that use functions with more flexibility than the straight line, such as the spline fit, will have little calibration bias but require relatively noise-free data. An aberrant point can usually be identified visually if the data reduction system allows graphic display of the data with the interpolated standard curve. Model-based calibration curves that fit the data well are less sensitive to one discrepant point since the curve is determined by minimizing the sum of the squared distances between the line and the response at each calibration point. The standard deviation of the estimate will identify noisy data or a discrepant point when it is clearly elevated compared with previous SD values. The same empirical or physical model will not always fit data from all types of immunoassays. Although the four-parameter logistic model works well with many immunoassays, it cannot be expected to fit all data. The increasing use in immunoassay systems of monoclonal antibodies which have homogeneous binding constants may lead to more specific models based on physical principles (Raab, 1983).

Software systems for immunoassay data acquisition and reduction are becoming more comprehensive. Extensive quality control systems capture data from replicate samples that can be used to weight calibration data when models are fit by least squares and provide comparison of new standard curves with previous data. The presentation of data in graphic form allows visual examination of data points with the fitted calibration line and is very useful with interpolative or model-based procedures.

APPENDIX A: BASIC PROGRAM TO FIT
FOUR-PARAMETER MODEL TO DATA
BY NONLINEAR LEAST SQUARES

The BASIC program shown here has been used by the author for many years to fit both radioimmunoassay and enzyme immunoassay calibration data. It has been optimized to fit the four-parameter logistic model, which is written in the form $y = a/(b + x^d) + c$ for this program, where x is the concentration and y is the response variable. On each iteration, two new values for the nonlinear parameters b and d are determined, and the linear parameters a and c are then determined by linear least squares. Thus starting values are required only for b and d, and crude estimates will suffice: d can be set equal to one (hyperbolic model), and b is set equal to one-half the highest concentration. On convergence, the program outputs values for a, b, c, d, the minimum sum of squares (Q), the standard deviation of the estimate, and R^2, which measures the variance in the response variable explained by the model. One is a perfect fit, and zero is equivalent to fitting a horizontal straight line through the mean of the response data. The program prints the estimated values of the response variables and prints the standards read off the fitted calibration curve. Unknowns can then be entered and their concentration calculated. Suggested exercises with this program include entering only four standards to see the almost "perfect fit" artifact discussed earlier and then entering five and six standard values. With good data, changing one point to an aberrant value should give an increase in the observed standard deviation of the estimate.

Example of Data: Radioimmunoassay of
Triiodothyronine (T_3)[a,b]

Counts	Concentration
10,020	0
9,123	0.5
8,078	1
5,666	3
3,541	8

[a]Concentration, nanograms per deciliter; response, counts per minute.
[b]$a = 27,160$, $b = 3.30515$, $c = 1813.45$, $d = 1.20961$, sum of squares $(Q) = 4227.84$, $R^2 = 0.99985$.

Point-to-Point Linear Interpolation

```
INPUT MODULE - 4P

10   DIM A(1Ø), F(4), X(2Ø), Y(2Ø), L(2Ø), Z(2Ø)

15   PRINT "ENTER (DEL-A OR CNTS); (-1) TO END"

20   H = Ø

25   FOR I = 1 TO 2Ø

30   PRINT "DEL-A OR CNTS =";

35   INPUT Y(I)

40   IF Y(I) < Ø THEN 87

45   PRINT "CONC =";

50   INPUT X(I)

55   L(I) = LOG (.Ø1)

60   IF X(I) = Ø THEN 85

70   L(I) = LOG (X(I))
```

```
75    IF X(I) < H THEN 85
80    H = X(I)
85    PRINT
86    NEXT I
87    PRINT "ENTER BØ, DØ (Y OR N)";
88    INPUT A$
89    IF A$ = "N" THEN 1ØØ
90    IF A$ = "Y" THEN 92
91    GO TO 87
92    PRINT "BØ";
93    INPUT BØ
94    PRINT "DØ";
95    INPUT DØ
96    GO TO 11Ø
100   BØ = H/2
105   DØ = 1
110   N = I-1
115   L1 = .ØØ1
120   B = BØ
125   D = DØ
130   GOSUB 1ØØØ
135   QØ = Q
140   GOSUB 5ØØØ
145   GOSUB 1ØØØØ
150   B1 = BØ + D3
155   D1 = DØ + D4
160   B = B1
165   D = D1
170   GOSUB 1ØØØ
175   Q1 = Q
185   IF ABS(D3/BØ) + ABS(D4/DØ) < .002 THEN 3ØØØ
```

```
190    IF Q1 < QØ THEN 2Ø5
195    L1 = L1 * 1Ø
200    GO TO 145
205    L1 = L1/1Ø
210    BØ = B1
215    DØ = D1
220    PRINT B1, D1, Q1
225    GO TO 135
3000   PRINT
3010   PRINT "A ="; A, "B ="; B1
3020   PRINT "C ="; C, "D ="; D1
3030   PRINT "Q ="; Q,  "SDEST ="; SQR(Q/(N-4))
3040   PRINT "R↑2 ="; 1-Q/(S4-S3 * S3/N)
3045   PRINT
3050   PRINT "sp sp I sp sp sp sp sp"; "Y", "YEST", "X", "XEST"
3055   PRINT
3060   FOR I = 1 TO N
3065   Z1 = A * Z(I) + C
3070   Z = A/(Y(I)-C) - B1
3080   IF Z < Ø THEN 311Ø
3090   PRINT I; "sp sp sp"; Y(I), Z1, X(I), EXP(LOG(Z)/D1)
3100   GO TO 312Ø
3110   PRINT I; "sp sp sp"; Y(I), Z1, X(I), "IMAGINARY"
3120   NEXT I
3130   PRINT
3140   PRINT "DEL-A OR CNTS";
3150   INPUT Y
3160   Z = A/(Y-C) - B1
3170   IF Z < Ø THEN 32ØØ
3180   PRINT "CONC ="; EXP (LOG(Z)/D1)
3190   GO TO 313Ø
```

```
3200    PRINT "CONC ="; "IMAGINARY"

3210    GO TO 3130


        SUBROUTINE 1000 - 4P

1000    S1 = 0

1010    S2 = 0

1020    S3 = 0

1030    S4 = 0

1040    S5 = 0

1050    FOR I = 1 TO N

1052    Z(I) = 1/B

1053    IF X(I) = 0 THEN 1070

1060    Z(I) = 1 / (B + EXP (D * L (I)))

1070    S1 = S1 + Z(I)

1080    S2 = S2 + Z(I) * Z(I)

1090    S3 = S3 + Y(I)

1100    S4 = S4 + Y(I) * Y(I)

1110    S5 = S5 + Z(I) * Y(I)

1120    NEXT I

1130    A = (N * S5 - S3 * S1) / (N * S2 - S1 * S1)

1140    C = (S3 - A * S1) / N

1150    Q = 0

1160    FOR I = 1 TO N

1170    W = Y(I) - A * Z(I) - C

1180    Q = Q + W * W

1190    NEXT I

1200    RETURN


        SUBROUTINE 5,000 - 4P

5000    FOR I = 1 TO 10

5010    A(I) = 0
```

```
5020    NEXT I

5030    G3 = Ø

5040    G4 = Ø

5050    FOR K = 1 TO N

5052    Z = Ø

5053    IF X(K) = Ø THEN 5Ø7Ø

5060    Z = EXP (D * L(K))

5070    F(1) = 1 / (Z + B)

5090    F(3) = -A * F(1) * F(1)

5110    F(4) = F(3) * Z * L(K)

5140    A(1) = A(1) + F(1) * F(1)

5150    A(2) = A(2) + F(1)

5160    A(3) = A(3) + F(1) * F(3)

5170    A(4) = A(4) + F(1) * F(4)

5190    A(6) = A(6) + F(3)

5200    A(7) = A(7) + F(4)

5210    A(8) = A(8) + F(3) * F(3)

5220    A(9) = A(9) + F(3) * F(4)

5230    A(10) = A(10) + F(4) * F(4)

5235    S = (Y(K) - A * F(1) - C)

5240    G3 = G3 + S * F(3)

5250    G4 = G4 + S * F(4)

5260    NEXT K

5265    A(5) = N

5270    RETURN

        SUBROUTINE 1Ø,ØØØ - 4P

10000   LØ = 1 + L1

10005   L2 = LØ * LØ

10010   Z = A(2) * A(2) - A(1) * L2 * A(5)

10015   X2 = (A(1) * LØ * A(6) - A(2) * A(3)) / Z
```

```
10020   Y2 = (A(1) * LØ * A(7) - A(2) * A(4)) / Z

10025   X1 = (A(5) * LØ * A(3) - A(2) * A(6)) / Z

10030   Y1 = (A(5) * LØ * A(4) - A(2) * A(7)) / Z

10035   R = A(3) * X1 + A(6) * X2 + A(8) * LØ

10040   S = A(3) * Y1 + A(6) * Y2 + A(9)

10045   U = A(4) * Y1 + A(7) * Y2 + A(10) * LØ

10050   T = A(4) * X1 + A(7) * X2 + A(9)

10055   Z = S * T - R * U

10060   D3 = (G4 * S - G3 * U) / Z

10065   D4 = (G3 * T - G4 * R) / Z

10070   RETURN
```

APPENDIX B: BASIC PROGRAM FOR POINT-TO-POINT LINEAR INTERPOLATION

This short BASIC program illustrates simple linear interpolation. The back slashes represent multiple-line statements. To see the effect of interpolation bias, enter an immunoassay standard curve into this program and observe that the concentration at the mean response of two consecutive calibrators is the mean concentration of those two calibrators. Compare these results to the four-parameter model fitted by nonlinear least squares and calculate percent bias.

Point-To-Point Linear Interpolation

```
5 L$="CONC.<LO STD." \ H$="CONC>HI STD."

10 PRINT "ENTER LO TO HI RESPONSES"

20 PRINT "NO. OF STDS."; \ INPUT N

30 FOR I=1 TO N

40 PRINT " ENTER (RESPONSE,CONC.)"; \ INPUT Y(I),X(I) \ PRINT \ NEXT I

50 IF X(1) >X(N) THEN T$=L$ \ L$=H$ \ H$=T$

60 PRINT "*****UNKNOWNS*****"

100 PRINT "RESPONSE="; \ INPUT Y

110 IF Y<Y(1) THEN PRINT L$ \ PRINT \ GO TO 100
```

```
120 IF Y>Y(N) THEN PRINT H$ \ PRINT  \ GO TO 100

130 FOR I=1 TO N

140 IF Y>=Y(I) THEN 160

150 GO TO 170

160 NEXT I

170 Y1=Y(I) \ X1=X(I) \ Y0=Y(I-1) \ X0=X(I-1)

180 X=X0+(Y-Y0)*(X1-X0)/(Y1-Y0)

190 PRINT "CONC.=";X \ PRINT \ GO TO 100
```

REFERENCES

Burden, R. L., Faires, J. D., and Reynolds, A. C. (1978). "Numerical Analysis." Prindle, Weber & Schmidt, Boston.

Raab, G. M. (1983). Comparison of a logistic and a mass-action curve for radioimmunoassay data. *Clin. Chem.* **29,** 1757–1761.

Rodbard, D. (1971). Statistical aspects of radioimmunoassays. *In* "Principles of Competitive Protein-Binding Assays" (W. D. Odell and W. H. Daughaday, eds.), pp. 204–216. Lippincott, Philadelphia, Pennsylvania.

Rodbard, D. (1974). Statistical quality control and routine data processing for radioimmunoassays and immunoradiometric assays. *Clin. Chem.* **20,** 1255–1270.

Rodbard, D., and McClean, S. W. (1977). Automated computer analysis for enzyme-multiplied immunological techniques. *Clin. Chem.* **23,** 112–115.

Rodbard, D., Lenox, R. H., Wray, H. L., and Ramseth, D. (1976). Statistical characterization of the random errors in the radioimmunoassay dose–response variable. *Clin. Chem.* **22,** 350–358.

Chapter 6

Immunoassays: Quality Control and Troubleshooting

Marie T. Perlstein

Division of Drug Metabolism
Ortho Pharmaceuticals
Raritan, New Jersey 08869

Part A: Quality Control: A Simple, Cost-Effective Approach

I. INTRODUCTION

Quality control (QC) is an essential function of every laboratory, and, when applied in a sensible fashion, it can be the most valuable tool a laboratory has. It is an objective means of measuring one's assay systems against the clinical requirements of the test. Specifically, a QC system is designed to ensure that results are within acceptable limits of accuracy and precision. In simple terms, a quality control program should help answer two very important questions: Are today's results reliable? and: Can we perform the same reliable results? Beyond these two practical necessities of life, quality control will help unravel the "mystery" of how assays perform and eliminate the unwanted element of surprise from laboratory routines.

This article will focus on a general overview of some of the basic elements of quality control and provide some simple, cost-effective ways to maximize QC data.

149

II. IMPLEMENTING A QC PROGRAM

Begin by examining the components of a typical immunoassay as it is performed in the laboratory, with particular attention to the concentration ranges that have the most critical clinical significance. What impact does each component have on the end result, on the other components? How can QC analysis help you find out? A quality control program should routinely assess equipment performance, reagent integrity, technique, assay conditions, and sample handling to provide a measure of the overall quality of the results.

As a starting point, look at your laboratory and your work load. Do you routinely rotate technologists, or do the same individuals run the same assays regularly? Is your testing population largely outpatients, or acutely ill inpatients? What tests do your perform? Are they of a critical nature, with a narrow range, or are they simply screening tests? The answers to these questions will help you to set sensible standards for your laboratory.

Selection of the control sample as well as the number of controls run for each test can influence the overall cost and quality of the results being generated. As a general rule, a control sample should be placed at concentration ranges where decisions are made that affect the clinical significance of the test result. With this in mind, it is possible to eliminate controls that fall outside the conically useful areas of the test. For example, including a very high level control in a serum folate assay may be unnecessary, since there is no clinical significance associated with elevated serum folate levels. Keeping the number of control samples used for each test to a minimum saves the cost of reagents and the time and effort to

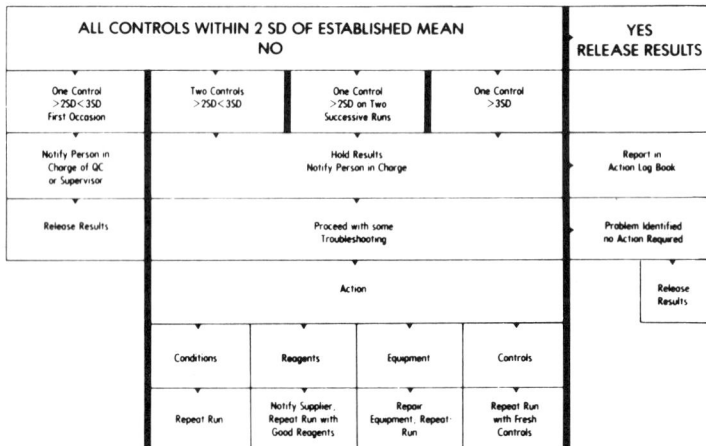

Figure 1. Scheme developed for a typical hospital laboratory using a two-sample quality control program with a ±2 SD range. The flowchart shows possible routes of action when one or both of the quality control samples fall outside the established 2 SD range of the mean.

track the data generated by extraneous controls. In addition, the statistics used in a two-control versus a five-control system are much less complex. An example of a flow scheme used to handle a simple, two-control system is shown in Fig. 1.

III. SELECTION OF APPROPRIATE CURVE FITS FOR IMMUNOASSAY DATA

The curve-fitting programs that are available for immunoassay data vary considerably in the way in which the data are manipulated. These variations occur as a result of the limitations associated with the sophistication of the hardware used for the system. The more elaborate desktop computers allow the programmer many options in designing the software so that the data can be processed at the speed necessary to maintain a timely flow of results. The less sophisticated versions cannot quickly process certain mathematical procedures that are necessary to compute coefficients and exponents needed to multiparameter models used in spline and logistic fits.

Therefore, some compromises are made and for the most part are unnoticed by and insignificant to the user. There are, however, circumstances where there is an inappropriate combination of data and curve fit that will allow the introduction of artifacts in the final results. It is essential that the mathematical manipulations used to fit the data do not skew the final calibration curve and introduce problematic artifacts. This can occur with poorly matched software and data that does not conform to the mathematical model used in the curve fitting program. Safeguards are generally built into software to avoid such hazards as hooks and tails that can happen with spline fits. The hooks and tails in the calibration curve make it possible to have two concentration levels that correspond to the same response. There are other more subtle ways in which inaccuracies can occur through poor data fitting. Therefore one needs to know as much as possible about the software package and the performance characteristics of the dose–response curve. To begin, let us look at the steps in transforming immunoassay data.

A series of calibration plots illustrates the progression from simple counts bound versus dose to a linear transformation through three steps. Figure 2A illustrates the relationship between the response (cpm bound) and the dose in a typical immunoassay. It is the simplest way to calibrate an assay. However, as the reagents age (especially the tracer) the assay tends to lose sensitivity. To normalize this effect, we can plot B/B_0 as a response parameter as shown in Fig. 2B. The dose–response curve still maintains a curvilinear shape and therefore requires advance programming to provide an accurate fit. Figure 2C shows B/B_0 plotted against the logarithm of the dose. This method transforms the curve from a hyperbola into an S shape. A further extension (Fig. 2D) transforms the data to

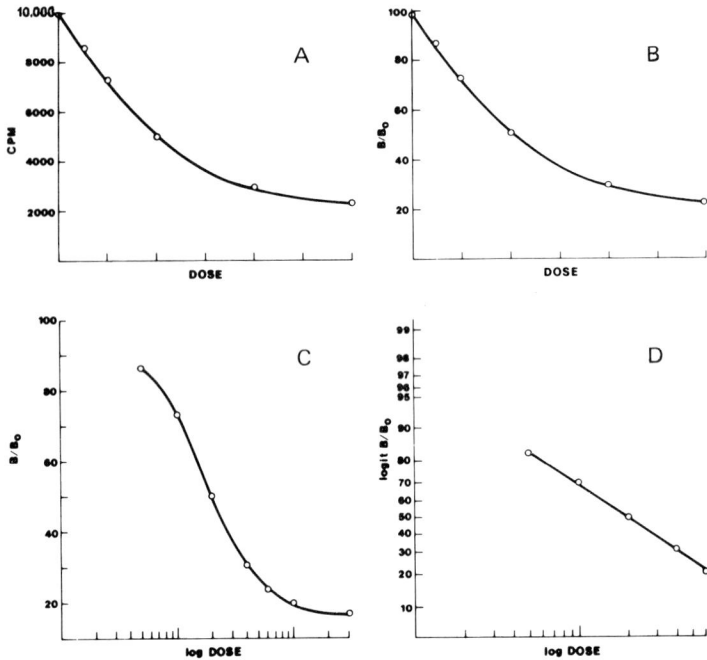

Figure 2. Curves depicting the transformation of RIA standard curve data. (A) Shape of the dose–response curve in Cartesian coordinates with the raw counts per minute on the y axis and the dose on the x axis. (B) The same data, but with B/B_o as the response parameter. (C) The data when B/B_0 is plotted against the logarithm of the dose. (D) Logit transformation of the B/B_0 versus log dose data and its effect in linearizing the curve.

a linear relationship by plotting the logit of the response versus the logarithm of the dose.

$$\text{logit} = \log \frac{B/B_o}{1 - B/B_o}$$

This is a popular way to treat immunoassay data since linear regressions can easily be programmed. A straight line is familiar, lends itself to visual inspection, and also provides a slope and intercepts, which may be used as indicators of assay performance.

In just three steps, then, it is possible to go from the natural dose–response to a straight line that can be used to calibrate the assay. However, whenever assay data are subjected to such mathematical manipulation, the new, derived dose–response relationship may obscure problems that would be apparent in the natural dose–response data analysis.

These indicators may be plotted and tracked on Levy–Jennings plots so that any deviation is readily apparent. In this way there is sufficient evidence available to attest to the correctness of the answers generated.

It is often useful to plot the data manually in a variety of ways. Visual inspection of manual plots can frequently reveal areas where the assay may lose sensitivity, and under these circumstances it may be wise to use a less extensive standard curve (e.g., eliminate the highest or lowest standard). These plots can be prepared from laboratory data generated in-house or from package insert data. After inspecting the manual plots, test the data on the software.

In selecting a data reduction algorithm, it is important to test the accuracy of the data fit. An inappropriate combination of assay characteristics and software can introduce bias into the results.

The simplest indicator of how well the data and software are matched is found in the comparison of the actual and calculated dose of the standards. As a rule, this difference should be within the expected precision for the assay at various dose levels. If the two values coincide, the data fit is acceptable. If, however, there is a wide variance between the values throughout the concentration range, another data fit should be sought because the results, or unknowns, may be skewed. This distortion can have an impact on the normal range and is sometimes the cause of poor performance in proficiency surveys.

Once the laboratory is confident that the fit and assay are well suited, monitoring the actual versus calculated dose can be used as a way to signal contaminated standards, pipetting errors, and so forth.

IV. EQUIPMENT

One of the most sensitive indicators of equipment performance is the precision of replicates. An increase in variation of raw counts is usually the first signal of equipment failure and is evident over the entire run. The more sensitive areas of the standard curve may not be as affected by poor precision of the replicates and the control, and the patient values (expressed in concentration units) may not reflect the same degree of imprecision. It may appear that only one of the controls is out of range, and it may take some time before a pattern develops, when, in fact, an equipment malfunction is present but unidentified. Therefore, inspecting the run for precision of raw counts can be a very valuable way to spot faulty tools.

Changes in equipment (Table I) can produce easily detected perturbations in results, such as inadvertent use of the wrong pipet. However, subtle differences can occur that may not be so apparent until you look for trends. A change in temperature or slowing of a centrifuge can affect precision, but you will need a history of your precision for this assay and this equipment over time to see it.

Table I. RIA Equipment and Precision Checklist

Item	Problem	Comment
Gamma counter	Loss in efficiency	Fewer counts will magnify error and compress the difference between the high and low standard, affecting assay range
	Contaminated carrier	Poor duplication; spurious results
	Contaminated crystal	Loss of resolution, causing change in slope, loss of assay range
Pipettes	Poor calibration	Uneven delivery of reagents may cause a change in maximum binding, total counts, and range
	Bad/wrong tips	Overall imprecision
Centrifuge	Change in temperature	May cause a change in the equilibrium point of the assay, affecting maximum binding
	Variation in speed	Poor pellet formation will cause imprecision
Water bath/incubator	Change in temperature	May cause a change in the equilibrium point of the assay
Test tubes	Wrong size	Poor mixing or evaporation creates imprecision
	Change in material	Change in hydrostatics may affect decanting efficiency
Mixer	Inefficiency	Poor suspensions, overmixed, denatured antibody
	Contaminated stirrer	Spurious results

Bad pipet tips can cause overall poor precision, as can an improperly calibrated automatic pipettor.

Even a change in the type of test tube used, say from polystyrene to polypropylene, can affect the results. In this case the hydrostatics of the interaction between the reagents and the tube wall may differ significantly and alter decanting efficiency.

V. REAGENTS

Immunoassays are complex, requiring several different reagents and a full standard curve to be performed each time the assay is done. This means that there are many things to watch and, on the other hand, many valuable bits of information contained in the standard curve. Figure 3 shows a scheme that may be used as a guide to reagent performance.

Many parameters are generated from the data management systems available for fitting standard curves. Perhaps the most universal is the ED_{50} (dose that corresponds to 50% maximum binding). This is steadfast, and causes for change in ED_{50} can usually be traced to the reagents or reaction conditions. For exam-

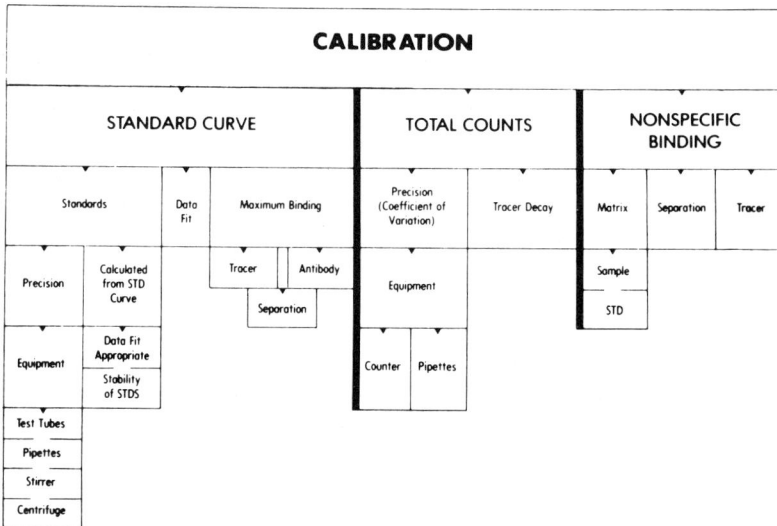

Figure 3. Flowchart illustrating the relationship of some of the information generated by the assay calibration and tracing possible sources of problems.

ple, an increase in antibody can cause an increase in ED_{50}, while a decrease in reaction time can cause the same effect. Therefore, if possible, keep a record, either a *Levy–Jennings* plot or a flat log, of the ED_{50} for use in suspect runs.

VI. ASSAY CONDITIONS

All assays are, to some degree, sensitive to pH, time, and temperature. Finding out to what degree an assay is sensitive helps to set reasonable guidelines for your laboratory. In beginning to assess an assay's sensitivity to reaction conditions, the first place to look is the package insert. Generally speaking, assays that work by a process of sequential saturation (reagents added in a step-by-step sequence) are extremely sensitive to time, while equilibrium assays are somewhat less so. Any assay that requires pretreatment of the sample, such as boiling, dilution, or buffering, merits special attention and should be watched closely for shifts in the daily mean or a change in nonspecific binding (NSB).

Since many assay protocols specify room-temperature incubation, it is important that the reaction be allowed to occur at specified temperatures. Laboratory temperature should be monitored and tracked daily and care should be taken that tubes are not placed on a sunny windowsill or directly under an air-conditioning vent during incubation. An environment that is too cold may decrease the range of the assay, and higher-than-normal temperatures may affect the maximum binding.

One reagent that is usually subject to less scrutiny than others is the control product. The assumption is that the quality control sample is perfect—identical to patient samples in matrix and analog of the analyte under study. However, this is not always or necessarily so. Commercial control products are derived from human or animal pools that have been spiked and subsequently freeze-dried. The laboratory then often divides the reconstituted control into convenient volumes, which are frozen and then thawed as needed. All of this manipulation can render the control less stable. In addition, small aliquots of samples stored in ''frost-free'' freezers can evaporate, giving results with an upward trend and leading the laboratory to question the entire assay. Home-made pools of patients samples can yield excellent control products but, being hand-crafted, may not contain stabilizers, so they too can show drifts and trends.

Before repeating a run because of suspicious control values, check the other facets of the QC program. If the calibration parameters are all within limits and the patient mean and spread appear acceptable, investigate the controls and use fresh ones in the repeat run.

VII. TECHNIQUE

Elimination of all technique-related errors in immunoassay is an ideal goal for most laboratories. Although this goal may never be totally attainable, it is possible to use assay-generated quality control information to identify and reduce technique-related problems. Reviewing data printouts immediately after a run is completed provides an opportunity to check on technique as well as equipment performance.

Although pipetting error is probably the most common technique-related problem, other seemingly minor occurrences—such as delayed or incomplete decanting—can affect precision and must be considered when coefficients of variation (CVs) begin to rise. On some occasions, however, a high CV need not cause great concern. This is related to the concept of heteroscadasticity—the inaccuracy inherent in the extreme ends of the curve. Also, in some assays the CV cannot be lowered because of the nature of the reagents or the procedure. Experience in running and tracking these assays will determine whether or not they provide clinically useful and reliable results.

VIII. PATIENT SAMPLES

Generally, the daily patient mean is remarkably constant. Aside from changes caused by samples at either extremely high or extremely low values, the daily mean can reflect how the specimens have been handled. For instance, a run might show the standards and controls to be functioning appropriately, but all the patient samples may be high (or low). In this event, suspect that the samples may have been collected in the wrong type of tube or drawn right after medication was administered, causing, for example, all *digoxin* results to be high.

In assays with boiling steps, samples may have been boiled too long or not long enough, producing spurious results. Microbial contamination of the samples or diluents can shift the mean results. It is important to consider all of the things that can affect any reagent when you begin to suspect a problem with the samples. For example, were the samples left out on a bench for a long period of time? What preservatives, if any, were used? Were the samples frozen and thawed? The answers to these questions can help to diagnose a problem in sample handling.

IX. CONCLUSION

Immunoassays offer many opportunities to monitor all aspects of assay performance, beyond just analyzing control sample results. Laboratories can cut costs, without compromising quality, simply by using the few sensible guidelines described here.

The basis for all QC, then, is to signal when things are right, as well as wrong, and lead those responsible for reliable results to the most likely sources of error *before* results become unreliable. Indeed, confidence in the quality of the results is the foundation of any clinical laboratory; and a sound, sensible quality control program is vital to engender that confidence inside, as well as outside, the laboratory.

Part B: Troubleshooting Immunoassays: Where the Practical and Theoretical Meet

I. INTRODUCTION

Troubleshooting immunoassays becomes necessary when all of the obvious causes of problems are ruled out and it is apparent that the more attention is needed to determine the source of a problem. This part describes several techniques for this purpose that go beyond the routine, casual examination of QC data.

II. PARALLELISM

Parallelism studies are a powerful troubleshooting tool for individual patient samples and can also be used to investigate changes in patient values that may result from changes in treatment of the samples.

The decision tree shown in Fig. 4 is based on simple serial dilutions of the suspect sample. The expected value in each dilution is calculated from the determined value on the undiluted sample and the dilution factor. The data are then plotted on plain graph paper with the found values on the y axis and the expected values on the x axis. Ideally, this should result in a straight line with a slope of one, an intercept of zero, and a correlation coefficient of 1.0. A variety of factors can cause a deviation from this ideal state, and they are indicated in the diagram.

Parallelism studies are very simple to perform and readily reveal the presence of exogenous materials in the specimen that render the specimen invalid for use with a particular set of reagents.

It is possible to detect cross-reacting compounds and matrix effects such as pH, salts, and endogenous binders that interfere with the reagents. The submission of an inappropriate sample type can be detected, because anticoagulants can cause disruptions of the binding kinetics in assays calling for serum samples (Fig. 5). Fibrin present in plasma can act as a source of nonspecific binding and its effect will also be apparent (Fig. 5). Therefore, the submission of an inappropriate sample can be detected. Dilutions of the suspect sample are made with the zero standard at 3/4, 1/2, 1/4, 1/8, and 1/16 of the original dose. The assay is performed on each dilution and the undiluted sample in the same run. The amount expected in each dilution is calculated from the value obtained on the undiluted sample and the dilution factor. There are several ways to express the data being tested for parallelism. The simplest method is to plot the amount of analyte found in each dilution on the y axis and the amount expected on the x axis. Usually, visual inspection of this comparison can quickly discern non-parallelism, and the response will fall in one of several possible patterns, shown in Fig. 5.

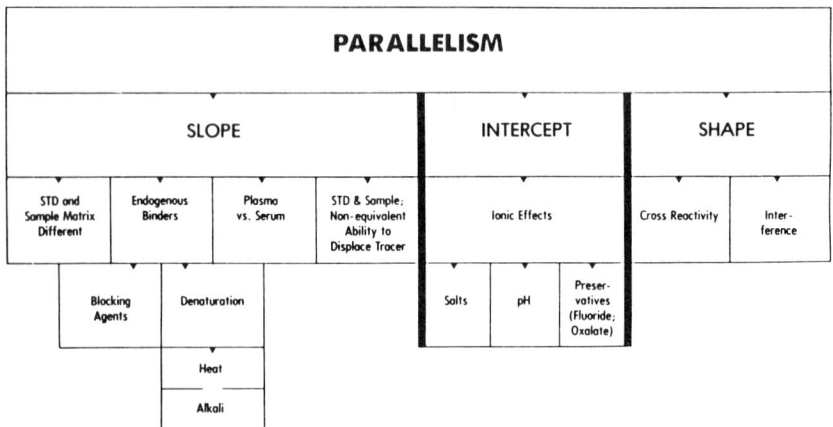

Figure 4. Flowchart summarizing some of the causes of nonparallelism and their relationship to the slope, intercept, and shape of the "Found versus Expected" plot.

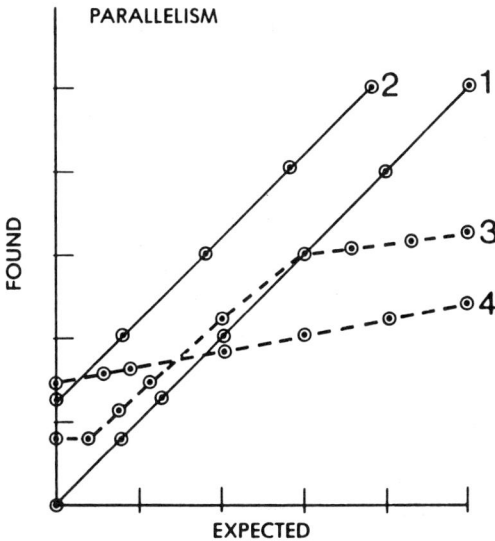

1 = Ideal
2 = Parallel, but may show a constant bias
3 = Effects of interferences such as salts, anticoagulants, pH,
that cause disruptions in binding kinetics.
4 = Non-parallel response generally due to endogenous
binders or cross reacting compounds present in the sample.

Figure 5. Types of curves that can result from parallelism studies. Curve (1) represents ideal data; curve (2) results when a linear, parallel relationship may be displaced by a constant amount; curve (3) shows nonparallelism usually due to interferences that cause disruption in binding kinetics; and curve (4) shows nonparallelism caused by something behaving as a binder for the analyte.

III. RECIPROCAL PLOT

Plotting the ratio of total counts to bound counts on the x axis and the dose on the y axis gives a linear response over a large portion of the concentration range. It has been shown that the slope of this line is equivalent to the binding site concentration and the numerical value of the y intercept (which is a negative number) is the tracer concentration. Therefore, it is possible to identify mistakes in the preparation and addition of the tracer and the antibody.

Nonspecific binding does not always remain constant over the entire concentration range, even when all else is the same. This effect has been attributed to the ability of nonspecific binders to play a more active role as the concentration of analyte increases, so that they can mimic the antibody reaction. Optimization of the separation system can be tuned to correct this problem. Changes or shifts in the region of concentration where the curve deviates from linearity and suspicious runs are characteristic of nonuniform nonspecific binding. Influences

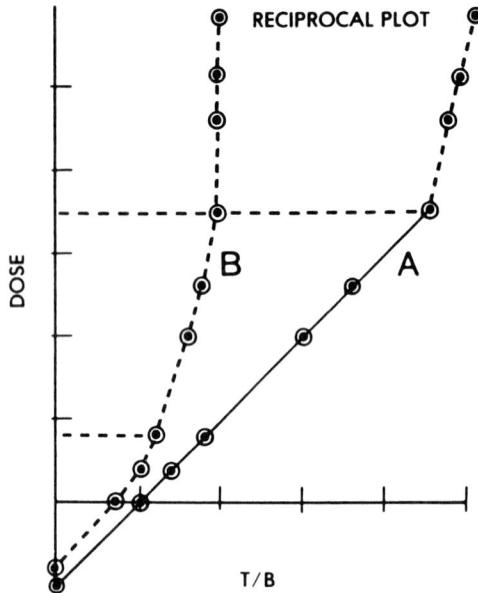

A = Data from acceptable run.
B = Data from questionable assay—showing characteristic
change in position nonlinearity when NSB is jeopardizing the
integrity of the assay.

Figure 6. Comparison of data transformed into a reciprocal plot for acceptable assay performance (curve A) and data from a questionable run (curve B).

on linearity include changes in the standard matrix, failure of blocking agents, and ineffective heat denaturation. Generally, this situation manifests its effect at higher concentration ranges and this type of data analysis can quickly sort out the problem. Examples of this are shown in Fig. 6.

IV. SCATCHARD ANALYSIS

The theory of radioimmunoassay (RIA) can be described by Scatchard analysis, which provides a way to compare data from different assay protocols on one coordinate frame. Scatchard analysis begins with the same raw data that are used for the assay-derived parameters and yields equivalent information, as seen in Fig. 7. In practical terms, the Scatchard plot and assay-derived parameters have a common basis and therefore are subject to the same influences.

Scatchard analysis can be a very useful tool for analyzing immunoassay data since it provides a way to look directly at events occurring in the assay tube. The

coordinates are calculated so that the assay may be evaluated at the m
level. From these data we can estimate the antibody affinity, binding ⌐.......
teristics, and concentration. Over time, the same assay procedure should yield
constant Scatchard analysis parameters unless one of the procedural variables
changes.

All immunoassays can be described by the law of mass action. With this as a
basis, Scatchard showed that a plot of bound counts/free counts (B/F) versus the
concentration of ligand bound gives a straight line, where the slope is equivalent
to the affinity constant of the antibody and the x intercept is proportional to the
concentration of binding sites. For a plot of B/F versus [ligand bound] to be
linear, certain criteria must be met:

1. Antibody and antigen (ligand) react in a one-to-one ratio in the simplest
way, that is without allosteric effects.
2. The separation of bound and free antigens is complete.
3. The system has achieved equilibrium.
4. The labeled ligand (tracer) and unlabeled ligand (standard or sample) behave similarly enough toward the antibody that the binding affinities of the
antibody toward each are within one order of magnitude.
5. The separation does not disturb the antigen–antibody complex.

It is rare that all of these conditions are met in an RIA. Therefore, there are
generally deviations from the straight line shown in Fig. 7, and Fig. 8 more
accurately represents a typical Scatchard plot from a standard curve.

The characteristics of the antibody have a direct practical impact on the performance of the assay. The behavior of the antibody binding (as described by the
affinity constant) can influence precision, dynamic range, maximum binding,
and minimum detectable dose. Scatchard analysis also provides a value for the

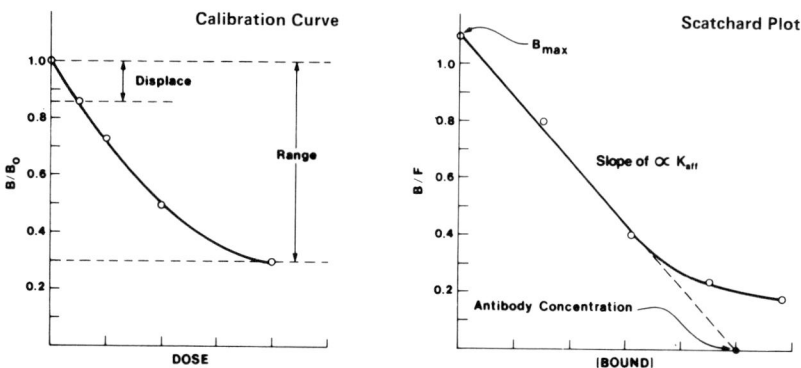

Figure 7. Relationship of the standard curve to the Scatchard plot. The curve on the left shows
standard curve data plotted as B/B_0 versus linear dose. The curve on the right shows some of the data
computed as B/F versus concentration bound in a Scatchard plot.

Representative Plots

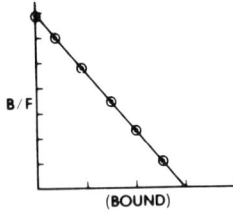

B/F

(BOUND)

IDEAL
All theoretical requirements met
Not often seen

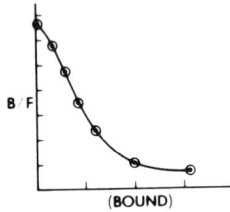

B/F

(BOUND)

TYPICAL for antiserum

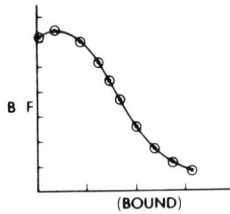

B F

(BOUND)

LOW DOSE HOOK
Allosteric binding: positive cooperativity
Damaged tracer

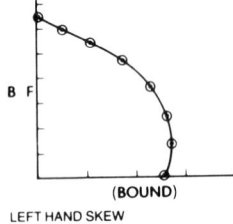

B F

(BOUND)

LEFT HAND SKEW

Comment

When examining Scatchard plots, we first look at the slope of the linear portion of the curve, which is proportional to the affinity constant of the antibody. This estimate of the K_a is influenced by the efficiency of the separation, the nature of the antibody, and the reaction conditions. When we examine the intercepts we can interpret the x axis as a function of the amount of antibody, which is influenced by separation technique and antibody dilution. The y axis is a function of the binding capacity, reflecting the B max, and is influenced by antibody-tracer affinity and the reaction conditions.

The overall curvature of the line may reflect the presence of multiple lower affinity antibodies in the antisera; and non-specific binding factors resulting from changes in a diluent for the standards or in the separation efficiency. Additionally, the curvature is a representation of the binding characteristics of the antibody which can affect the dynamic range of the assay.

The low dose hook effect is seen as a result of allosteric binding or damaged or out of date tracer. The presence of a low-dose hook negatively affects low-end sensitivity.

A left hand skew is a sensitive indicator of assay conditions, i.e. time, temperature and pH that have the greatest impact on the state of equilibrium. The presence of a skew affects the high end of the concentration range and is often associated with high non-specific binding.

Figure 8. Various characteristic assay problems which distort the Scatchard plot.

concentration of binding sites, which is a direct measure of the amount of antibody present. Similarly, a change in the amount of antibody will affect the maximum binding (x intercept). The product of the affinity constant K_a and concentration of binding sites is often referred to as the binding capacity of the reagents and can be determined from the y intercept of Scatchard analysis.

Scatchard analysis is a very useful troubleshooting tool which can pinpoint problems in addition to confirming suspected reasons for trouble. Valuable information can be derived from the shape, the slope, and the intercept of the linear portion of the curve.

The slope of the linear section of the curve is equivalent to the affinity constant (an intrinsic property) of the antibody, which determines the ratio of bound to free fractions at equilibrium.

The affinity constant should not change. However, a number of experimental factors can alter the reaction conditions so that the antibody behavior may exhibit an apparent change. Thus, in addition to the introduction of a different antiserum, the affinity constant of the same antibody may apparently change due to differences in reaction milieu (pH, salt concentration, matrix) and conditions (time and temperature).

The separation system can have the effect that the data generated will show alterations in the computed affinity constant. Poor separations generally have effects that are evident in the higher dose ranges and cause the curve to "peel" away from linearity sooner than it does with efficient separation. It also is possible for a robust charcoal separation to strip the tracer from an antibody, giving the impression of lowered antibody affinity. When second-antibody separations are used, the concentration or titer of the second antibody (Ab^2) must be adjusted carefully; insufficient or excess second antibody will not give a good immune complex, and an apparent decrease in the affinity constant of the primary antibody (Ab^1) will be observed. This effect can be minimized by the use of polyethylene glycol (PEG), which causes both soluble and insoluble complexes of Ab^1–Ab^2 to precipitate. Stoichiometric equivalence of Ab^1 and Ab^2 is not required. Since PEG can also precipitate serum proteins, changes in the PEG reagent can give rise to different changes in nonspecific binding of the standards, controls, and patient samples that may not be proportional in each medium.

The concentration of antibody binding sites is proportional to the x intercept and can be estimated in extrapolating the linear portion of the Scatchard plot. The presence of lower-affinity antibodies in addition to nonspecific binders in the matrix causes the curve to deviate from linearity. However, all of these factors should remain constant in their overall influence on a given assay. Changes in intercept then are due to a mistake in antibody addition (either first or second antibody). This effect will also be present in the maximum binding well, and the combination of alterations in B_{max} and the x intercept is diagnostic of inappropriate antibody concentration.

The shape of the Scatchard plot is influenced by the overall combination of antibody concentration, antibody affinity, integrity and concentration of tracer, standrad purity and matrix, separation efficiency, stage of equilibrium, and the molecular interaction between the antibody and the ligand.

Index